HOW I LOST A 100 POUNDS!

My Personal Weight Loss Strategies for Optimal Health and Happiness

EMMA GREEN

Book

1

CONTENTS

FOREWORD

"I love everything about Emma's connection to weight loss and health."

Hi, my name is Nat Lee, and I've spent most of my life looking pretty good and feeling great. That was up until I started eating on the run and allowing my busy life as a mom to take hold of me. While working too.

In truth, I knew I should eat great food, but time constraints and "motherly craziness" got the better of me. I made sure my son ate well. But I didn't, which was silly, really. Parenting is one of those things that just takes over your life, I suppose. So, anyway, I kinda ate loads of stuff I shouldn't, and drank sodas and milkshakes an awful lot. Chocolate and takeout became my best friend, and I became overweight, by anyone's standards. No one really told me I looked bad, I mean, most people aren't that obvious. But when I was diagnosed with a severe illness and bedridden for four years, it became time to do something to help my recovery. I made the change as soon as I could.

Since reading Emma's books, I've lost 18.5 kg (which is 40 amazing pounds). And I've managed to keep it off by following her wonderful advice, and by using her awesome, easy-to-do recipes. I live relatively simply, but her guide to nutrition and her tips and tricks have helped me a bucket load. Thank you Emma, you've literally changed my life!

ACKNOWLEDGMENTS

I would like to take the time to personally thank my mother and father for their immense dedication and support that went into getting this book out and into the world, including its editing. I would also love to thank Justine Sherwood for her excitement in helping me bring this wonderful, life-changing book to life, through thorough planning and organizing of the information, herein. Her long talks and influence throughout my journey have been simply heartwarming. A warm and special thank you also goes to the amazing Dr. Stephen T. Chang for his extensive guidance and knowledge of dieting as an incorporative practice. I would also like to thank Jim Baker, Louis Fraser, and Annie Tolson for much guidance and commitment in aiding the content for readers of my book. Last (but not least), I would also like to send a big shout out to Dean Lawson for helping me to get the whole idea hatched and off the ground so it could be shared in a larger format, and on a platform sufficient enough to help more individuals to succeed in their own journeys. And, to everyone else who gave me insight, support, love, and guidance for my book, I thank you from the bottom of my big, open heart. I cannot describe the depth of my gratitude to you all. Without your love and support, it would not have been

possible to make this a reality. Thank you so very much. Love
Emma xx

Chapter One

MY STORY

Hey everyone! I'm so glad to be able to share my story on how I lost 100 pounds! I think the best way to tell you how I lost so much weight is to start off by telling you the story about my journey, and how it

all came to be, from start to finish. Then, that way, you can get a better understanding of how everything happened and how I overcame my own obesity problem. A BIG one. Before I begin, I want you to know that I am not a doctor, a dietician, a naturopath, or a scientist. And so, the information I give to you is the result of what I did to get my own personal achievements and results, thus far. However, please also know, that the information I give to you is definitively backed by science, scientific results, major studies and that it is also backed by many health professionals, doctors, naturopaths, and dieticians, too. Please always seek advice if you are unsure. Each body reacts differently to processes, exercise, and foods.

So, "Hi," my name is Emma Green and I was born in the lucky year of 1984. Yep, born and bred in sunny West Virginia... yup, you heard it correctly - I'm from the highest-ranking obesity state in the entire country, unfortunately. And I can tell you that I am really disappointed to see that this is the case. In truth, as a state, we have an ongoing love for deep fried food here, and we are definitely not shy about it. As a child, I remember the food well. I have memories of sugary biscuits, the best barbecue fried chicken in the whole (entire) world, loads of different cheeses, and my mom's famous (very naughty) pecan pie. I loved all of these things, and food became my major, most pleasurable treat in life.

In all honesty, I lived in a semi-poor family, and we couldn't afford the "right" clothes or any of the expensive cool stuff, and so I was picked on at school and developed social anxiety at a very young age. I ate for comfort, and I guess my problem started when I was around 15 years, or so. This was coupled with the fact that Southerner's diets include loads of big, deep fried foods, barbecues, carb-loaded treats, and a plethora of sugary desserts. Also, because the weather is not as temperate in our state, it's hard to exercise outdoors for most of the year. In reality, it's just too damn hot! And there really aren't that many opportunities for in-state exercises during the months when it's boiling hot, either. On really hot days, it can get up to over 80 degrees Fahrenheit. Our average temperature is around 65 throughout the year.

Growing up, I learned to love my southern lifestyle. It was cheaper to eat badly than it was to get fresh produce at the time. We didn't have heaps of money and we got by as best we could. So, my mom got what was cheap when we ventured to the local store. The food was inexpensive, and my mother made us the best meals, despite us living below the poverty line. When you're poor, you tend to eat more calorie-dense foods because they're actually cheaper than fruits and vegetables, and that's just how it was for us. I don't blame Mom for spoiling me, because, in reality, she didn't know any better. The only difference nowadays, is that we are noticing the effects that modern day (westernized) diets have on the body as a whole.

From the age of 15, I started to stack on the weight, severely so, and I also suffered from an extreme case of social anxiety. I remember feeling completely closed off from the rest of the kids at school. Not only because of my weight, but because I was quite shy and nervous to mix with others. I don't really know why it occurred. Anyway, over time, my lunchbox became a place I felt drawn to. Because Mom was in there, and she was my biggest safety net and supporter. All the little treats and pieces of food were like heaven to me at that time. And, as my lunchbox grew, so did I. Unfortunately.

After a time, I got diagnosed with arthritis. I think the arthritis was diagnosed between 27 and 28 years of age, from memory. It was a major pain in the neck, quite literally. I had excessive knee pain and standing for long periods was excruciating, some days. It took so long sometimes, to do even little things. The pain was unbearable in my back as well. I also loved to cook, but everything ached so much at times, that even that was hard to do. The news literally shocked me when I heard it. The experience of it sucked more than I can put into words. I was in pain most days, more than not. A symptom of my obesity, so I was told. The pressure in the body from taking up the excess load became a real nightmare.

By the time I turned 29, it had gotten to the point where I had constant joint pain nearly every day, and my self-esteem became nonexistent. I was depressed, and my blood pressure was up to the roof. My doctor said I was on my way to heart disease, and that I was lucky not to have diabetes yet, however, at this rate it was inevitable, he said. My mother and father both had diabetes and I think the real turning point in my life was when my auntie Mel had a stroke that very same year. She lived through it, however, but she never really was the same after that. At the time, it really shook me seeing her like that. And, I definitely knew that it could easily be me. She had to be hand fed and couldn't talk properly. It was so very sad.

As it turned out, I had been doing everything back-to-front and upside down. I had been exercising without paying attention to my diet or any nutritional needs at all. I'd tried multiple brands of "skinny" pills, and had been riding a stationary bike for hours on end (with marginal results). I tried everything... Yep! I even starved myself with diets that gave temporary results. The stress of doing all of it with little to no results made me feel absolutely hopeless, worthless, and more than overly annoyed! I felt like completely giving up, many times. On so many occasions, in fact. I was lost and felt like I couldn't find my way out of it. I nearly gave up! Semi-depressed was my state of mind. It felt like everything sucked. I was very sad, mad, and exhausted.

I remember clearly the summer of 2015, a blistering 95 degrees Fahrenheit, one hot day. I was crazily trying to look for answers and I was scanning the net for anything that would help me. I remember being so desperate as I was looking through pseudoscience cures because everything I'd done had failed. I read that this herb would cure this, and this lotion would stop this pain, and one site claiming it was the "must-have" cure for all, while another touting its adverse effects. Gosh, it was all conflicting and very confusing. And then, by chance, I stumbled onto a book called, "The Tao of a Balanced Diet - Secrets of a Thin and Healthy Body." The main concept stated that what you put into your body becomes a part of your body. If you put in healthy food, your body becomes healthy. If you put in "garbage," your body becomes "garbage." Giving me an easy-to-understand wealth of knowledge, and real practice methods of eating the right things, in the right way. Skeptical as I was, I had nothing to lose, so I ordered the book - and within 4 days it was in my hands. This book would become the main catalyst for my view on how diet plays into the role of not only your weight loss, but gaining health and happiness in the process.

This knowledge I added to everything else I'd learned and studied beforehand, and then I put it all into action. It took me 22 months to do what I did. I added it all together and I literally lost over 100 pounds!!!! I did it safely, properly, and successfully. Without starving myself, exercising ridiculously, or feeling hopeless eating salad... all day long. I really did it!! And now I want to help you too. I can't wait, actually! Ready... I am... let's go!

Throughout this title, we're going to cover the fundamentals of weight loss, including nutrition, weight loss myths, keto and paleo diet styles, superfoods, herbs, the importance of quinoa, juicing, green smoothies... and much, much more! Inside you will get an insight on nutrition with regard to dieting and the definitive role it plays in weight loss as a major, staying factor. You will also come to understand the importance of water weight and how you can help yourself by sticking to one, mind-blowing, game-changing rule. There are recipes included throughout the title, and some other wonderful tips and advice, as well! So, let's start by looking at some of the U.S. statistics our country is facing as a whole. After that, we'll get stuck into how to lose weight, safely and effectively. Ready? Good! Let's go!

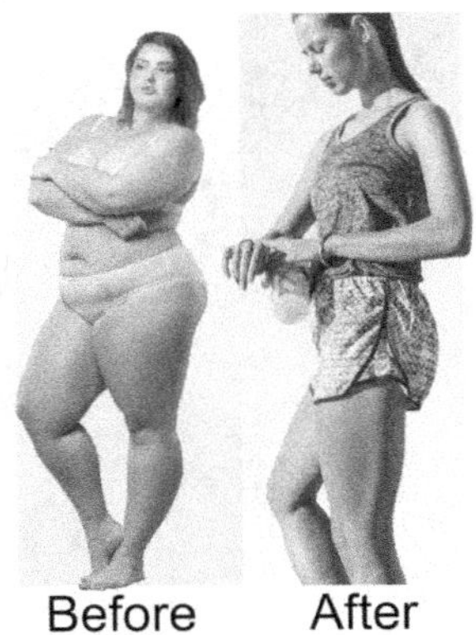

FREE GIFTS!

Here are 3 bonus books I want to gift you for coming and reading this title! Sign up to my newsletter and you will receive:

Weight Loss Myths - 9 myths that you are mostly likely doing right now that are totally pointless and are a waste of time toward your weight loss goals.

How to Lose Weight Fast – A 10 day plan I personally put together to make that weight literally melt before your eyes (it worked for me!)

And... Weight Loss Secrets - Secrets the main stream media and health industry never talk about because (let's be honest) things that work don't make them money!

Click here to sign up! or for paperback versions grab it through the ebook completely FREE!

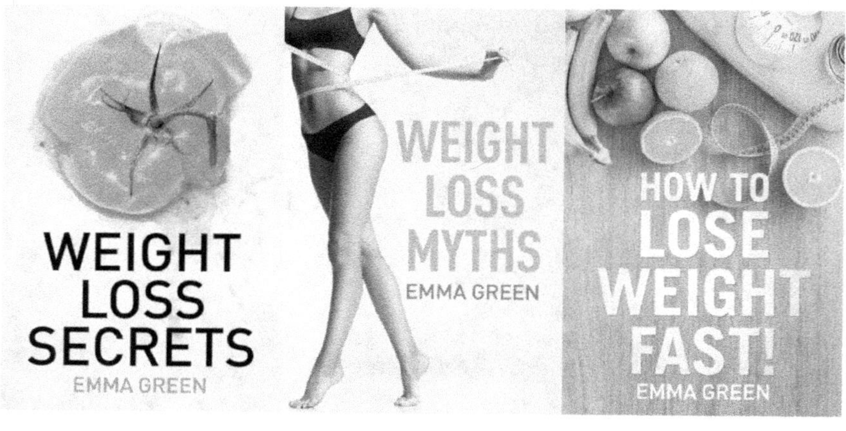

Chapter Two

U.S. STATISTICS SHOW OBESITY IS RISING

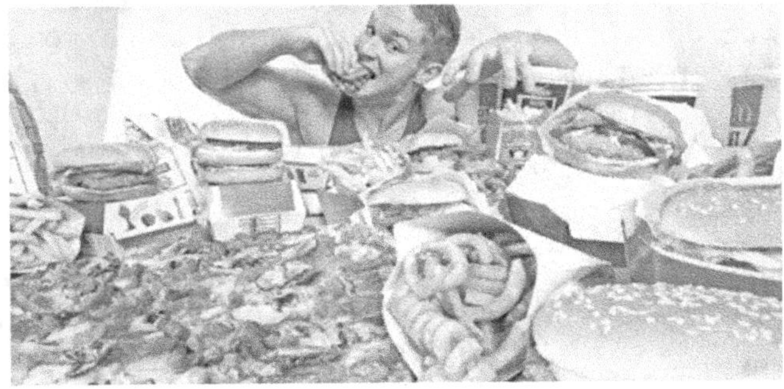

It's clear that obesity in the U.S. right now is a significant problem, and it is an issue that shows no signs of slowing down, unfortunately. Recent studies have definitively confirmed the trend in the number of Americans who are both overweight and obese. This number is growing each and every year, and has been for the past three decades.

One of the latest studies that was conducted by the Center for Disease Control and Prevention shows: **that almost 40% of adults in America are obese.** What is even more alarming, is that the study showed a figure of **nearly 20% of U.S. adolescents are also obese.**

These numbers are, in fact, the highest figures ever recorded and appear to get worse with each survey that is conducted.

Long-term health (which is associated with these figures) is troubling because it shows that **one in five children from the age of 6-11 years is obese**; as is the statistic that shows **one in five children aged 12-19 years is, too.** These are mind-blowing statistics. If this isn't bad enough, the study has also shown that **one in ten preschool-aged children are also obese, not just overweight.**

SO, WHAT IS OBESITY?

The medical term for an individual who has a body mass index of 30, or above is known as obese. The findings from these latest studies in the U.S. further support reports from the World Health Organization that show childhood obesity around the world is also a growing problem, and one that has **increased by tenfold over the past forty years.** Wow, these statistics are both sad and shocking.

When children become obese or overweight, the chances are they will stay in this state and will be exposed to higher chances of dying earlier during adulthood. We need this to change. Now!

WHY ARE SO MANY PEOPLE OBESE?

The Department of Agriculture made a report that showed that **the average American consumed around 20% more calories per year than they did in earlier years**. Much of this comes with the increase in meat consumption. These days, Americans consume a figure of around 195 lbs. of meat, compared to a value of just 138 lbs. during the 1950s.

The increase in meat consumption means an increase in added fats that are consumed, with figures rising by two thirds over the same period of time. This coupled with the lack of necessary exercise, means that individuals have gained weight definitively. In that 40 years, grain consumption in America has grown by 40% as an additional leverage factor.

Another one of the main contributors to the rise in obesity is fast food. This is directly related to an individual's body mass index. **An average American diet consists of around 11% of fast food, alone**. With this, comes **loads of added sugars from soda and energy drinks**, and other processed additions, which wreak havoc on a person's waistline. Not to mention the **overload of calories** found within each meal.

Chapter Three

WEIGHT LOSS MYTHS

Before moving to the diet section, there are a few myths you might have heard, and these described are most-definitely false. Let's take a look at them so we can get clearer.

MYTH #1 ALL CALORIES ARE EQUAL

In essence, a calorie is a unit of energy, and that much is definitely true. However, how these calories or "units of energy" affect your body is very different, indeed. Varying foods pass through various metabolic pathways and affect hormones that regulate body weight and hunger.

A good example of this, is consuming 100 calories of chocolate. This would have a much more significant (and negative) impact on your body than 100 calories worth of healthy salad. Additionally, a protein calorie is not the same as a carb or a fat calorie. The body utilizes the vitamins and minerals in certain foods differently. So, we need to stay with foods that boost vitality, and also aid in weight loss, not fat storage, as an ideal necessity.

MYTH #2 YOU WILL SEE WEIGHT LOSS EVERY DAY

This is not true, some days you will go up a little, and other days you will drop down again to compensate. This is one reason they say not to weigh yourself each and every day. In the case of women, they might have more water retention during their menstrual cycle, so be aware of that.

MYTH #3 SUPPLEMENTS WILL HELP INDIVIDUALS TO LOSE WEIGHT

Most supplements, especially when studied against their claims of weight loss, are shown as not as effective as their claims make out. Most people fall for marketing, and they fall under a placebo effect where they are conscious of what they eat as a result. It's usually not due to the product being viable, though. So, a "quick fix" is usually not the real deal, unfortunately.

MYTH #4 CARBOHYDRATES WILL MAKE YOU FAT

It is a fact that low-carb diets will help you to lose weight, and they can do so - without a dramatic reduction in calories. As long as you keep carb intake low and protein consumption high, you can lose weight, but it will take time. Not all carbs are equal, actually. It is true that refined carbs like sugars and grains are linked to obesity, but whole-wheat carbs are, in fact, healthy.

MYTH #5 FOODS LABELED "DIET" WILL HELP YOU LOSE WEIGHT

Many types of junk food are portrayed and marketed as being healthy. These include gluten-free foods that are processed, fat-free foods, and low-fat foods, as well. They appear healthy from the labeling, yet the actual ingredients tell a very different story. Some are loaded with preservatives which the body cannot use effectively, if at all.

When you count your calories, and you have reduced them, don't be tempted to cut them even further, because you will feel hungry, and you might become very irritable. And that doesn't help the cause; not at all. The one advantage of the ketogenic and paleo-styled diets as part of your goal-reaching, is to make sure you feel satisfied, and that you are able to resist the urge to eat "other" non-viable foods.

Chapter Four

HOW TO LOSE 10 POUNDS IN A WEEK

Now, you must be thinking, how on earth can someone lose that much weight so quickly? I mean, that's just not possible. However, once you understand how, it's surprisingly easy to do. Depending on how much you weigh, I've known people who have lost over 20 pounds in their first week of implementing such strategies. But you need to understand that you will be losing water weight, not fat. Losing that much fat in such a short time is impossible, and it's not the least bit healthy in the slightest. We will discuss this in this current chapter, and the causes of water weight, too. We'll do this; including the negative impact it plays on your body, and we'll also learn how to know if you are retaining water and cellulite - the byproduct of water retention.

1. Let's first identify if you have water retention. If you have cellulite, then 100% (without a doubt) your kidneys are not functioning right. To check for cellulite, check your buttocks, thighs, belly, and upper arms for jelly light tissues underneath the skin.

2. If you experience rapid changes in weight (such as 5-6 pounds in a

day or two), then that is definitely an indication of water retention. No fat can come or go that quickly.

4. If you press down on your leg or arm for a second, then withdraw it, you will see a white impression, briefly. That's how you know you have water retention. If you are not retaining water, there will be no white mark, or it will go away immediately. The longer the white impression stays, the worse the retention in the body.

The kidneys in the body have the function of filtering waste water from the blood. A lot of how much water the kidneys are capable of filtering out relates to the effectiveness of your kidneys' performance for this task.

Contrary to popular belief, healthy kidneys can filter (on average, for men and women) **6 cups of liquid in any twenty-four-hour period**, and if they are pushed to filter larger quantities than this, they become **overworked** and will **weaken**, over time. We were always told 8 cups, however this is gravely not the case, and it can cause many health issues, actually.

If you have healthy kidneys and you consume six cups of water/liquid (maximum) per day, you will be on a level that is **conducive to health**. However, if you drink more than this (and what your kidneys can efficiently handle), this fluid remains in the body and travels back around the bloodstream. It can only be eliminated through perspiration. Up until that time, it stays in the body and will be carried around as **excess weight**. This is not something we want, for two main reasons: great health and weight loss achievement.

As you have set your goal to lose weight and stay healthy during the process, and because you have to embark on a lot more exercise for the duration, perspiration will not be a problem. Because you might only lose a proportion of the water levels inside your body, any incoming water or fluids will back up the levels, and they become retained in the skin. When there is enough buildup of water, the skin bloats so it can accept this water (that is ready to be released through perspiration).

There are two ways that cellulite can be reduced and removed, the first and **simplest way is to reduce your fluid intake (drink less) to stay at the balanced six cups, or slightly less, per day.** For the whole process, this is the most critical part.

The second step is to **stimulate these cellulite deposits and break them up.** Two of the most comfortable ways of doing this are by having a **hot bath or by taking a sauna**. Massage the fatty areas whilst in or under the heat.

So, yes, the best way to get rid of these deposits is to heat them up and break them down. In simple terms, **the more they are massaged, the more they will break up and can then be eliminated.** This helps the fatty deposits to break up. Once you do this (while the body is hot), the pores will open and allow for a much more significant amount of perspiration too.

MAKE SURE YOU UTILIZE THE 6-CUP (PER DAY) RULE

When people are trying to lose weight by whatever means, there is a good chance they cut out the junk foods. They might even have a salad for dinner, accompanied by a glass of water, as an example. This is fine.

However, this can lead to a miscalculation of water intake as salad contains water too, which has to be purified by the kidneys. When 6 cups of water (or any other liquid) per day is the maximum, **this includes anything that might hold water.**

Fruits, vegetables, soups, and any other beverages all go toward this total count. It is a little hard to calculate when you consume foods which contain water, and this is another area where juicing and green smoothies can come to the rescue. Essentially, because you can measure these - so the liquids in the fruits and vegetables can be accounted for as part of your daily "6 cup" intake.

Let me be clear though, if you do a rigorous job or play rigorous sports in which you sweat a large amount, then that is fine to drink over the 6-cup rule on that given day. Remember, weight loss is the goal of this chapter but not at the sake of dehydration and passing out. We want to do it safely. Always.

So, now that we understand the why and how, we can begin to reduce the water within our body. The easiest is obviously as stated above; to reduce further intake of water to our normal kidneys' filtering level. 6 cups a day. For this, (to remove the already present water) you must do activities that make you sweat, and the ones that come to mind straight away are: saunas and steam rooms. Relaxing and losing weight at the same time, what a dream that is... a surprising reality, in fact! Try to get into these as much as you can; the more the better. Also, limit the time in them for 10-15 minutes. Massaging the cellulite will remove this over time, however, please know that many toxins and poisons reside within the cellulite, so only massage small parts slowly each time. If you do too much too quickly, you can actually poison yourself.

There are many, many other things you can do in conjunction with these steps, and to lose the weight very rapidly, and if you want to know more about the actual methods involved, please check out my book, "How to Lose 10 Pounds in a Week," in which you will learn: 7 day weight loss plan, how to use the right nutrition that makes your body a fat burning machine, tips to aid water retention and toxin prevention, how to (once and for all) negate the myths surrounding weight loss, how to understand that you no longer need to work out crazily in order to shed pounds, and the addition of some awesome recipes to get you started on your all-important journey. This title also includes some real ideas on what you don't need to do with regard to weight loss, including the best methods for overall success! Click here! It's completely FREE for Ebooks!

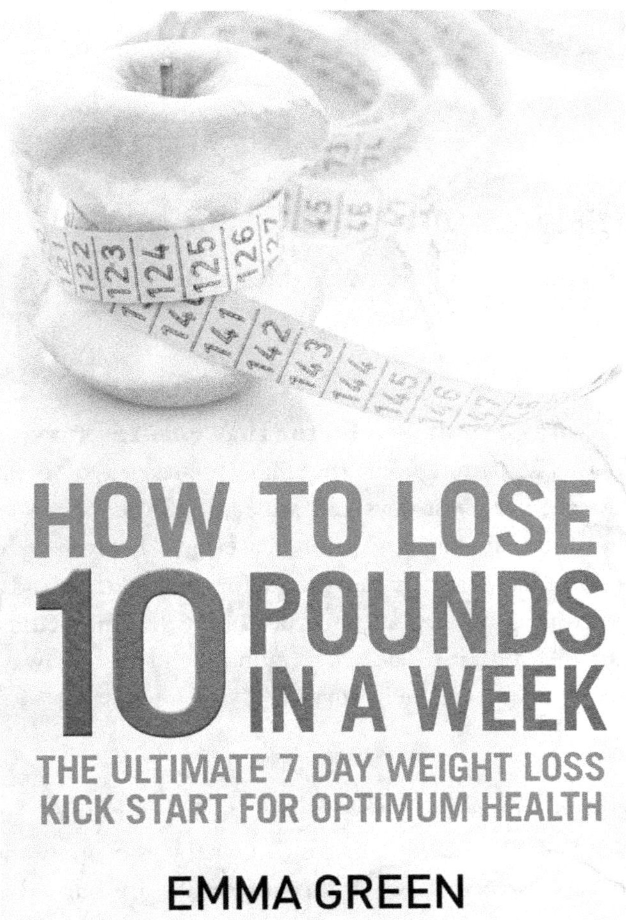

Chapter Five

HOW TO LOSE BELLY FAT FAST (FOR MEN AND WOMEN)

THE SCIENCE BEHIND THOSE EXTRA POUNDS

So, now we will see how the body stores these stubborn fat deposits, and what it is using that fat for.

Storing fat in the body is a factor that ensures survival. It has been this way all throughout the many centuries of evolution. It started from the very first days and was nature's way of protecting the body during food shortages. Although we have evolved by countless thousands of years, and it is rare to go for extended periods without food and becoming hungry, **the human body still has this defense mechanism.** And so, it processes food in much the same way as it has always done. It likes to make us survive.

Fats are also known by the name "triglycerides," and when these are consumed they are broken down by the body and passed around the bloodstream. It is at this stage they are burned as energy (or stored as fat reserves) for future use.

When this fat is ingested, it actually becomes stored into fat cells by the name of adipocytes, and these cells are located all around the body under the layer of skin with a high number of them deposited in the abdominal region of the body - unfortunately.

So, when this fat is not burned for energy, it is stored continually until the time when the body needs energy reserves. If a current state of overeating and lack of exercise ensues, then this leads to an inactive lifestyle which then leads to the body's metabolism becoming slower. And so, there is less requirement for it to burn these fat deposits.

TWO TYPES OF BELLY FAT?

There are, in fact, two types of fat around the midsection. The first is **visceral** which surrounds our internal organs and the second is **subcutaneous** which is that podge that we love to grab and squeeze! Well, that we "used to" love to grab and squeeze.

Now, with these two fats, the one that surrounds the organs is visceral, and it's actually the one that is easier to deal with. This can be rectified by a healthier diet and taking up exercise. Subcutaneous fat is the type that causes the most problems and is the one that is most difficult to lose. It is this one that leaves us with the unflattering "love handles" and "beer bellies" that so many adults are blessed with.

A VICIOUS CIRCLE

If it was just these that caused problems, it might be easier to cope with and reduce those extra pounds around the belly. But... nature has one more surprise up its sleeve for all the dieters out there.

When the body is stressed, hormones are released from the adrenal glands. These being cortisol, norepinephrine, and epinephrine. When you first become stressed, that's when it's time for these hormones to come into play.

Norepinephrine passes signals to the body to halt the production of insulin, and so you can have a larger supply of fast-acting blood glucose for when it is needed. Next, epinephrine relaxes the muscles in the abdominal region muscles and intestines while (at the same time) reducing the blood flow to these. Once the stressor has passed, it is the job of cortisol to tell the body to stop these other two hormones being produced, and return to its normal functioning and digest again, normally.

LOSING BELLY FAT – TIPS AND TRICKS

- **Utilize a lower calorie intake per day 1200 (women) and 1700 (for men).**
- Utilize a **keto and/or paleo-styled eating plan.**
- Maintain the balance in nutrition (**Five Element Theory**), as discussed later in this title.
- **Avoid "junk" foods** that are processed, loaded with salt and sugar, and full of chemicals.
- **Drink distilled water,** or rain/filtered water. Never drink tap water.
- Use **juicing/green smoothies** to accelerate metabolism and to add to the nutrient boost for the body.
- Utilize the **stomach rubbing technique**. Lay on your back; place palm on navel; rub clockwise from center, in small circles and then expand until the upper and lower sections are being rubbed. Now, reverse the movement until you get back to the center again, in an anti-clockwise rotation. Move slowly and use light pressure only. This is an ancient Chinese (Taoist) technique.

- **Limit your fluid intake to 6 cups per day** (including the fluid found in foods).
- Add **chrysanthemum flowers** for additional success, in the form of a natural (sugar-free) tea. These are great for weight loss.
- **Exercising less strenuously** is more productive for belly fat removal.
- **Bike riding for 15 to 20 minutes daily** helps the metabolism to increase.
- **No abs or crunches** should be done, because weight loss needs to be achieved first, in terms of total body weight. This occurs before belly fat loss is accomplished.

LET'S DISCUSS SOME OF THESE POINTS FURTHER:

THE KETO DIET

The keto diet consists of a low-carbohydrate intake, a moderate inclusion of proteins, and a high level of fat consumption. By doing this, the body will enter a state we know as ketosis. This state efficiently produces ketones in the liver compared to glucose which is created from carbs and transported around the body. Ketones replace glucose and bring many health benefits for the body, along with a high reduction in body fat, thus aiding weight loss up to three times faster than a more conventional diet.

PALEO DIET

The paleo diet often goes by the name of the "Caveman Diet" for the simple reason you can consume anything you wish that can be hunted or gathered. This includes leafy greens, veggies, nuts, meats, and fish as main staples. Anything that is processed or man-made is prohibited as it falls outside the rules of what the diet aims to achieve. Because everything is fresh and healthy, calorie counting is not a necessity so there will be no feeling of not being satisfied at meal times. The other advantage is it's a great diet when looking to lose weight, because your body only consumes healthy nutrients and vitamins.

JUNK FOOD

This is the term that is given to any food that contains high levels of calories which come from added sugars and fats. These are unhealthy because they contain small amounts of fiber, vitamins, nutrients or proteins. Junk foods can also include high protein foods which have been prepared using saturated fat. To simplify what this is, it is the majority of foods that you can purchase from fast food outlets or "packet foods" in grocery stores. All these junk foods are directly linked to obesity and help individuals to incur a higher risk of heart disease.

DISTILLED WATER BENEFITS

Due to the composure of distilled water, it is the purest form of water you can get. All of the impurities are removed; which is much healthier for the body. One other benefit, is its ability to help flush toxins from the body better than tap or bottled water. Although these waters might have a better taste than distilled water, this is not to say they are any better for you. This taste comes from impurities or inorganic minerals that have been added to help purify the water and make it safe for drinking. I do not recommend them.

JUICING/GREEN SMOOTHIE BENEFITS

Juicing and green smoothies are beneficial because they include all of the fruits or vegetables that they are made from. A green smoothie includes everything and can be assimilated by the body with no need for digestion to take place, in comparison to when these nutrients can usually become lost through cooking. Green smoothies also allow you to increase your healthy intake of raw vegetables that can help with detox as well as weight loss. It helps to cleanse the liver and also promotes healthy skin.

CHRYSANTHEMUM TEA BENEFITS

This tea has been shown to bring many health benefits that are only just realized by the western world. Being used for thousands of years in China, and mostly used in Chinese medicine to help with increasing blood flow which helps with heart disease, and improves the body's resistance to insulin. And this is great because it helps to aid in weight loss. Toxins and heavy metals can also be flushed through the system which allows the liver to perform its functioning, without becoming overloaded. The tea has also been used extensively when mixed with other green teas to produce a high-fat burning tonic.

SMARTER CARDIO

Although cardio can do the body some good, it can have an adverse effect if you are aiming to lose weight. Cardio places the body under exercise stress, which it is unable to differentiate from any other form of stress. Due to the way the body functions, it tries to preserve fat because it thinks the body will need reserves for later. This then means your body burns energy from lean muscle tissue rather than burning any fat reserves. It is healthier and more beneficial to undertake an exercise that uses a broader muscle base that will burn more calories rather than become exercise stressed. Exercising by bike riding for 15 to 20 minutes per day is advised, instead. The other tips will be discussed later in this title including the Limiting the liquids you consume per day, and more.

For further information on losing belly fat, check out my amazing book, "How to Lose Belly Fat Fast for Men and Women." It contains great information on the right nutrition that's vital to succeed throughout your weight loss journey, problematic exercise types that you don't need to do, the prevention of water retention issues, foods and drinks to avoid at all costs, the importance of PH and the five elements of food, and other great tips you'll need to boost your overall success in your learning and implementation. Included are also some

great recipes you can use to get started! Click here! Another
FREE Ebook!

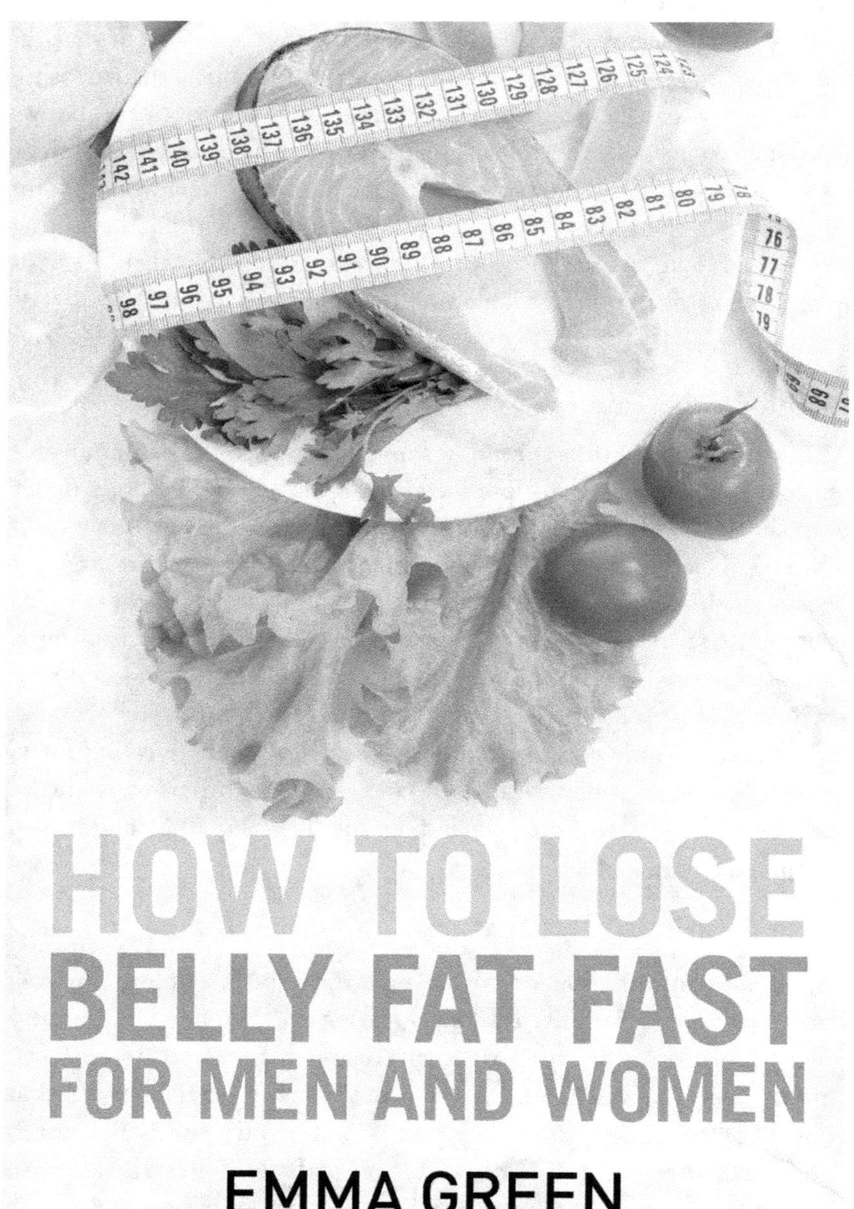

Chapter Six

THE IMPORTANCE OF KETOGENIC AND PALEO-STYLED DIETING

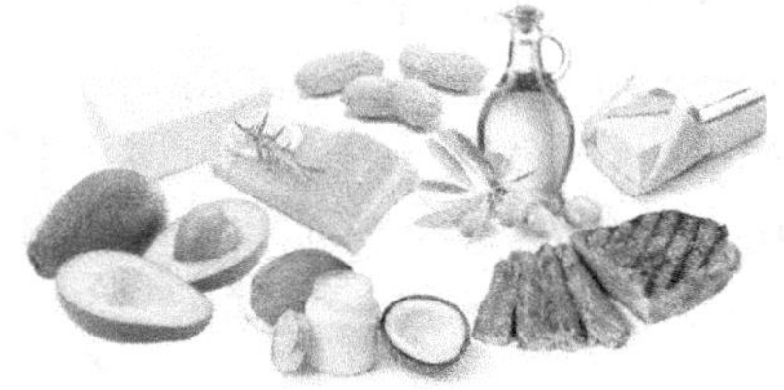

UNBELIEVABLE KETO:

I loved keto because I could eat real, wholesome foods. Including meat which is packed full of iron and protein. I love steak, so this worked well for me and I didn't ever feel hungry. At the end of this chapter I'll be sharing some ketogenic recipes – my most favorite ones, so you can enjoy them too!

The keto diet is a way of eating which promotes ketosis in the body, and to do this correctly, you follow the following ratios in your meals for the day:

Percentage of Low Carbohydrates – **5% (or lower)** of your daily calories will be made up of carbs.

Percentage of Moderate Protein – **Between 15% and 35%** of your daily calories will be made up of protein.

Percentage of High Fat - Between **60% - 80%** of your daily calories will be made up of fat.

When you follow these ratios, something magical really happens. Your body is depleted of glucose, and it ramps up its production of **ketones** which are then used to **produce energy**.

KETOSIS

Let's understand this process. This is where the energy for the body comes from the ketones that are produced, compared to the glucose (sugar) which usually provides the energy. It is the westernized, modern diet that provides us with high carb foods and leaves our bodies in a state of glycolysis which is, in fact, bad for us. The ketogenic diet negates this high carb state, altogether.

WHAT ARE KETONES?

Ketones are the source of energy that your body will use when it's going through ketosis. They are produced by the liver when glycogen levels are very low. These ketones are a fuel supply which burns lower inside the body.

KETO AND INSULIN

This is the absolutely magical part of the keto connection. When you are on a high carb intake, your body produces high amounts of insulin which help to carry the glucose around the entire body. In this state, fat deposits stay as fatty deposits and then they build up over time.

When you are in a state of ketosis, your body breaks down these fat deposits in the liver to convert them to ketones, which are then used as the body's primary energy source. Not only does this help you to lose weight faster, but your insulin levels remain at a stable level rather than peaking and dropping throughout the day. So, this helps to maintain the energy. This then also makes it much harder for your body to store any extra fat.

KETOGENIC AMAZING DIETARY BENEFITS

Weight Loss – This is the number one reason people follow a full-fledged keto diet. The body quite literally changes into a fat-burning machine.

Increased Energy Levels – The body prefers to use ketones as an energy source if it can. You have more energy throughout the day rather than in peaks and troughs.

Lessened Hunger Pangs– You will find you are less hungry when you follow this great eating plan.

Cholesterol – Contrary to what was said in the past, the keto connection will actually help to lower cholesterol levels. Recent studies are showing this more and more.

Diabetes and Blood Sugar – the keto diet type has been shown to have a positive effect on diabetics and blood sugar levels, overall. Many studies support this fact. To aid credibility to the diet, many studies have shown positive, long-term effects in participants. In one study conducted by the NCBI, patients showed a decreased body mass index and a decrease weight over 24 weeks. Triglyceride levels also showed a significant decrease after 24 weeks and blood glucose also had the same effect. No major side effects were shown in patients and the diet was deemed a success, for both safety and sustainability.

AMAZING PALEO:

Let's look at paleo as a great style type too. The paleo "mantra" is widely known as **no grains, no beans, no dairy, no sugar, and no industrial seed oils**. So, it literally supports the keto style, as well.

I love paleo because it's super easy to remember the rules. I put the mantra on my wall and I eat whole foods like beetroot and fish which are two of my favorites. I felt so much better not eating things from a packet that were loaded with sugar and salt. I noticed the change within a week, and I could eat great meals without starving myself.

SO, WHY THE PALEO?

The focus should be on vegetables, lean meats, fish, chicken, and eggs. Fruit and nut consumption is kept to a minimum when on the paleo diet. Full fat products are allowed, and aren't calorie controlled.

THE MAJOR BENEFITS OF THE PALEO DIET INCLUDE:

- Major weight loss over time
- Crushing of inflammation within the body
- Helping in disease prevention
- Can fully eliminate some diseases
- No calorie counting required
- Utilizes whole, non-processed foods
- Uses whole foods requiring less energy to digest
- It has similar benefits to the Mediterranean diet
- Scientifically proven to aid health, overall
- Cardiovascular health improvements can be seen
- Effective in treating inflammatory bowel disease
- Effective in treating metabolic syndrome

LONG-TERM DIET RISKS CAN BE COUNTERACTED:

- Compromised bone health through lack of calcium (which can be utilized elsewhere, in vegetable intake, as an example)
- High fish consumption (if toxins are present) can cause a build-up of toxins

SO, HOW DOES THE PALEO DIET WORK?

The easiest way to understand the paleo (or paleolithic) diet is to realize that the predominant consumption of food is to utilize **whole** foods. **Whole foods can be described as... foods that have not been processed or redefined (with additives or artificial substances and chemicals).**

The paleo diet avoids dairy products, grains, sugar, legumes, processed oils, excess salt, alcohol, and coffee. The ideas behind the diet are **founded by Walter Voegtlin** and have been popularized by many dieticians and chefs very widely, and around the entire globe.

The paleo diet style works to promote health, long-term. And, on a cellular level, it maneuvers food ingested, and in doing so, it begins improving the body's composition and its overall metabolic effects by way of substances taken in. A noticeable comparison to the high sugar/high salt diets profoundly demonstrated in the westernized culture. In fact, the paleo diet offers a wonderful alternative to the "dangerous" westernized diet, on the whole.

One recent study by Diabetologia (in 2007) showed that patients were significantly improved in terms of glucose tolerance after remaining on the paleo for 3 months. The median range of weight loss was 11 lbs. In a timeframe of 12 weeks, a reduction of waist circumference was also seen at an average of 2.2 inches.

THE KETO-PALEO:

You can utilize both the ketogenic and paleo diets together, in fact, they complement each other in many ways. **They both have major weight loss benefit potential and are easy to understand and follow.** It's great when the magic happens, because your body's way of coping changes. It heals faster, and its metabolism responds more quickly, without the stress of coping as a mechanism. Everything you now put into it has a purpose... and then the weight loss can begin! Safely and effectively, may I add.

SIX GREAT KETOGENIC RECIPES: BREAKFASTS:

RECIPE#1: MARVELOUS MINI-KETO QUICHES

I love this recipe because I get to eat mozzarella cheese and it's super easy to do, too. It takes 30 mins and tastes so amazing!

Ingredients

- 14 eggs
- 3 plum tomatoes, diced
- 2/3 of a cup of mozzarella cheese torn into bite-size pieces
- 1/3 of a cup of cheddar cheese, grated
- 1/3 of a cup of white onion, diced finely
- 1/3 of a cup of pickled jalapenos, sliced
- 2/3 of a cup of salami, diced
- 1/3 of a cup of heavy cream
- 1 pinch of sea salt and black pepper, to taste

Instructions

- Preheat oven to 160 degrees C and lightly grease a muffin tin. Half fill any muffin trays with water.

- In a mixing bowl, beat the eggs.
- Add to the mixing bowl all remaining ingredients and mix well, then season with salt and pepper.
- Divide the batter into the muffin tins equally, and bake for around 25 minutes.
- Can be stored in the refrigerator and reheated before eating.

RECIPE#2: YUMMY SAUSAGE AND EGG WITH CHEESE

Eggs and sausages are two of my faves! Combine these two things together and it's heavenly. Time to cook is minimal too!

Ingredients

- 3 oz. of breakfast sausage
- 1 egg
- 1 tablespoon of olive oil
- 1 cheddar cheese slice
- chives or spring onion for garnish, chopped

Instructions

- Heat a small skillet over medium heat and add olive oil, cook sausage until no longer pink, and browned on all sides.
- In the same pan, cook the egg until the desired "doneness" is reached.
- Transfer to a serving plate and garnish with chives or green onion.

LUNCHES:

RECIPE#3: CHEDDAR AND HAM MAYO WRAPS

Again, I love cheese, and the mayo just oozes into the recipe. My type of yummy. I absolute recommend this one, it's quick and easy to do.

Ingredients

- 2 low carb wraps
- 4 to 5 tablespoons of mayonnaise
- 4 oz. of cheddar cheese, grated
- 4 oz. of sliced ham
- jalapenos or pickles, thinly sliced to taste
- sea salt and black pepper, to taste

Instructions

- Heat the skillet over medium heat, place wrap in a dry skillet and warm through for about 30 seconds.
- Take the warm wrap and spread the mayonnaise.
- Place ham slices on the wrap, and then sprinkle with the grated cheddar cheese.
- Add slices of pickle or jalapenos according to taste.
- Fold the ends inward and then roll tightly.

RECIPE#4: BLT MAYO WRAP WITH AVOCADO

Avocados are amazing. The flavors rock in this recipe, and are a great treat for friends too!

Ingredients

- 8 lettuce leaves
- 6 tablespoons of mayonnaise

- 12 strips of bacon
- 1 tomato, sliced thinly
- 1 avocado peeled, seeded, and thinly sliced
- 1 tablespoon of olive oil
- sea salt and black pepper, to taste

Instructions

- Heat a skillet over medium heat, add a dash of olive oil and cook the bacon to your liking.
- Wash and pat dry the lettuce leaves and then flatten slightly.
- Spread 1 tablespoon of mayonnaise onto each leaf.
- Season with salt and black pepper.
- Add 2 slices of bacon to each lettuce leaf.
- Divide the avocado slices and sliced tomato, and place onto each leaf.
- Wrap tightly.

Dinners:

RECIPE#5: ZESTED ORANGE STIR-FRIED BEEF

I love anything stir-fried. The flavors pop in this one, and are perfect if you want to impress that someone special.

Ingredients

- 1/2 a lb. of beef steaks, sliced thinly
- 1/2 a cup of low-sodium beef broth
- 2 tablespoons of coconut oil
- 1 medium onion, diced
- 1/2 an orange, for zest and juice
- 4 cloves of garlic, minced or crushed
- 2 inches of sliced ginger
- a good pinch of ground cinnamon

- 1 teaspoon of low-sodium soy sauce
- 1/2 a teaspoon of fish sauce
- 1 bay leaf

Instructions

- Slice beef into 1-inch thin slices.
- Heat a medium skillet over medium-high heat and add coconut oil.
- Add the diced onion, garlic, and ginger, and sauté for 1 minute.
- Add the beef strips and cook for 5 minutes and add the soy sauce and fish sauce.
- Add the beef broth, bay leaf, cinnamon, and orange juice.
- Increase the heat and cook until broth juice has begun to thicken.
- Transfer to serving plates and top with orange zest. Serve hot.

RECIPE#6: SHRIMP WITH SWEET AND SPICY CHICKEN

I love spice. The flavor permeates throughout the whole meal, and it's a nice change from the ordinary.

Ingredients

- 2 chicken breasts, boneless and skinless
- 20 large shrimp, peeled
- 1/2 a cup of mushrooms, sliced
- 2 large handfuls of spinach
- 1/4 of a cup of mayonnaise
- 2 tablespoons of sriracha sauce
- 1 tablespoon of coconut oil
- 2 teaspoons of fresh lime juice
- salt and black pepper, to taste
- 1 teaspoon of garlic powder
- 1/2 a teaspoon of crushed red pepper

- 1/2 a teaspoon of paprika
- 1/2 a teaspoon of honey
- 1 spring onion, finely chopped

Instructions

- Tenderize chicken slices between plastic wrap until it is of a 1-inch thickness.
- Season with sea salt, black pepper, and garlic powder.
- In a skillet over medium heat, add the coconut oil and chicken breasts.
- Cook for 8 minutes and turn once. Reduce the heat and cover.
- Add the sliced mushrooms to the chicken. Add oil if required.
- In a mixing bowl, whisk together the mayonnaise, sriracha, and honey.
- Heat a pot over medium-high heat, and place the shrimp in one layer.
- Add the sauce and toss to coat. Cook for around 3 minutes until the shrimp are pink. Stir occasionally to prevent burning.
- Remove from the heat and add the fresh lime juice and toss to cover all the shrimp.
- Divide spinach onto serving plates with cooked mushrooms.
- Add the chicken and shrimp, and coat with the sauce.
- Sprinkle with chopped spring onion to garnish.

For further information on losing weight on the ketogenic diet, please check out my amazing book, "Top 50 Ketogenic Recipes - Quick and Easy Keto Diet Recipes for Weight Loss and Optimum Health." Along with great recipes, we'll take a look at how keto works as a main player in weight loss and health, and we'll also take a look and see the major benefits that can be achieved through the use of this science-backed nutrition type. And, of course, 50 wonderful recipes you can use for breakfasts, lunches, and dinners! Click here! Ebook is Completely FREE! X

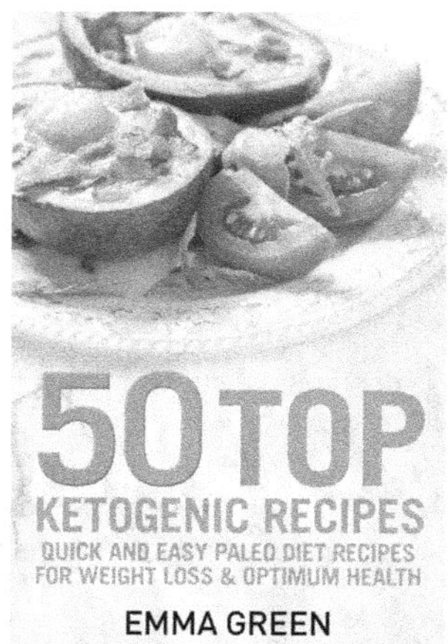

SIX AMAZING PALEO RECIPES: THIS IS QUICK, EASY... AND YUMMY TOO. I ALWAYS FEEL FULL AFTER THIS ONE!

BREAKFASTS:

RECIPE#1: HEALTHY "NO-OAT" MEAL

Ingredients

- 1 small handful of walnuts
- 1 small handful of pecans
- 2 tablespoons of flax seed (ground)
- 1/2 – 1 teaspoon of cinnamon (ground)
- 1 pinch of nutmeg (ground)
- 1 pinch of ginger (ground)
- 1 tablespoon of almond butter
- 1 banana (mashed)
- 3 eggs
- 1/4 cup unsweetened of almond milk
- 2 teaspoons of pumpkin seeds
- 1 handful of fresh berries (choose seasonally)

- 1 tablespoon of organic honey

Instructions

- Add walnuts, pecans, and flax seed with spices to a processor. Blend until it's not totally ground into powder form.
- Whisk eggs and almond until consistency thickens to a loose custard.
- Thoroughly blend the mashed banana and almond butter and add it to the custard, mixing well as you go.
- Stir in the nutty mixture.
- Microwave or gently warm on the stovetop.
- Sprinkle pumpkin seeds and berries on top.

RECIPE#2: SANDWICH BONANZA

Coconut changes everything! I absolutely love the flavors here. Great for entertaining too!

Ingredients

- 1 cup finely of ground unsweetened coconut
- 1 egg
- bacon
- mince patties
- bread

Instructions

- First you will need to make the coconut griddle cakes.
- Mix the fine coconut and the egg together.
- Cook on the stove like pancakes.
- Cook bacon and mince patties.
- Stack it in a sandwich.

Lunches:

RECIPE#3: ITALIAN VEGETABLE LASAGNA

I love anything Italian... so here's something Italian, need I say more?

Ingredients

• 700g lean mince meat

• 1 onion, diced

• 2 garlic cloves (finely chopped)

• 5 tablespoons of rich tomato paste

• 30 oz. of diced tomato

• herbs – parsley, sage, mixed Italian herbs, thyme, basil, cumin ground, cinnamon

• 1 eggplant, sliced

• 1/4 butternut pumpkin, sliced

• 6 zucchinis, sliced

• 3 tablespoons of olive oil

Instructions

• Preheat oven to 180 degrees Celsius, fan-forced.
• Make sauce by frying onion and garlic in a pan until brown.
• Remove from pan, by placing in a bowl.
• Now add and cook the mince.
• When the mince is cooked, return the onion and garlic to the pan adding the herbs (to taste).
• Now add tomato paste and cook for 3 minutes.

- Add the diced tomatoes and leave to simmer on low heat for 30- 45 minutes.
- Layer eggplant slices along the bottom of an oven proof dish. Layer eggplant with 1/2 the mince sauce. Now layer with pumpkin slices, spreading the remaining mince sauce over the pumpkin; then layer zucchini slices on-top.
- Brush olive oil over zucchini slices.
- Bake for 30-40 minutes.

RECIPE#4: TASTY MOROCCAN SKEWERS

Flavor-packed and great with any salad. If you want to impress, this recipe goes all the way!

Ingredients

- 8 wooden skewers; soaked in cold water for 30 minutes
- 3 chicken breasts, diced

Marinade

- 1 garlic clove
- 2 teaspoons of honey
- 2 tablespoons of lemon juice
- 1 tablespoon of oil
- 1 teaspoon of cumin (ground)
- 1 teaspoon of salt
- 1/2 a teaspoon of cayenne pepper
- 1 teaspoon of turmeric (ground)
- 1/2 teaspoon of cinnamon (ground)
- pepper to taste

Instructions

- Dice chicken into cubes

- Make marinade by combining ingredients in a small bowl, mixing well. Put chicken in a large dish, pour marinade over the top and coat well. Cover and leave in the refrigerator overnight.
- Preheat oven to 180 degrees Celsius.
- Thread chicken onto skewers and place on an oven tray lined with baking paper.
- Slowly pour marinade over chicken.
- Bake for 35-40 minutes or until chicken is cooked properly.

DINNERS:

RECIPE#5: PORK WITH HONEY AND APPLE

Pork and honey together... could anything be more exquisite? A delight to cook this one.

Ingredients

- 50g of olive oil
- 1/4 cup honey
- 8 x 1/2 lb. pork fillet (pieces)
- 4 pink lady apples, sliced horizontally into thin slices
- a pinch of chopped sage
- 3 bunches of spinach
- 4 tablespoons of pine nuts
- a squeeze of lemon juice
- salt and pepper

Instructions

- Preheat oven to 180 degrees Celsius.
- Combine olive oil and honey over a low heat until honey has

melted. Glaze the pork in the honey, dipping well, cooking both sides for around 3 minutes.

- Now, on a baking tray, lay out 8 groups of 4 apple slices (approx.) and brush with honey mixture, then add the sage and the pork.
- Top with 2 or 3 more apple slices and another coat of honey as required.
- Bake for 20 minutes, or until the apples have caramelized.
- Separately, (in a fry pan on low heat) place in pine nuts and stir until brown.
- Steam the spinach until cooked, and mix in a squeeze of lemon juice to taste.
- To serve, place pine nuts on top of spinach as a complementing side dish to the pork main.

RECIPE#6: PIZZA PALEO

Again, Italian anything rocks! And everyone loves pizza, right? Plus, it's so easy to do.

Ingredients

- 3 teaspoons of olive oil, divided
- 1 cup of almonds (ground) or other nut choice (to taste)
- 3 tablespoons of cashews (ground) butter
- 1/3 of a cup of egg white
- 1/2 cup of onion, chopped
- 2 cloves of minced garlic
- 1 chopped red pepper
- 1/2 cup of halved grape tomatoes
- 1 large Italian sausage, cut into 1/2" slices
- 1/2 cup of marinara sauce
- 1/2 teaspoon of oregano

Instructions

- Mix ground nuts, cashew butter, and egg whites in a large bowl.
- Grease a pizza sheet with 2 teaspoons of the olive oil, then spread the dough mixture over it, making a thick crust.
- Preheat the oven to 180 degrees Celsius.
- In a pan, add the remaining olive oil and the slices of sausage.
- Cook until brown, then remove the sausage once cooked.
- Add the garlic, the onions, and red pepper to the pan. Sauté the vegetables lightly, but not so they are too soft.
- Cover the dough with the marinara sauce, then add the meat and vegetables, excluding the tomatoes.
- Add the oregano, then bake for 25 minutes.
- Remove from oven, adding the halved tomatoes, and serve.

For further information please check out my helpful book, "Top 50 Paleo Recipes: Quick and Easy Paleo Diet Recipes for Weight Loss and Optimum Health." It also touches upon the unfortunate health issues from Conventional US-based diets, the benefits of paleo in weight loss and overall health, and (of course) the top 50 awesome recipes you can utilize for breakfasts, lunches, and dinners! Click here! Ebook is completely FREE!

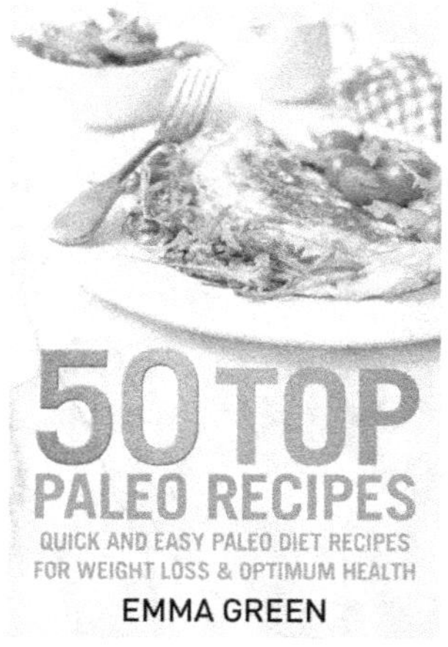

Chapter Seven

ADD QUINOA

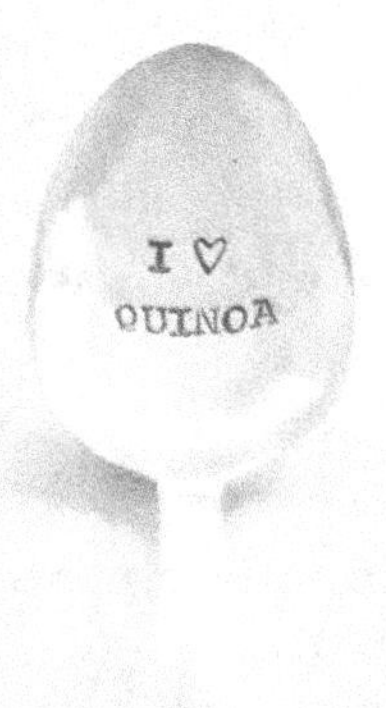

Quinoa is one of those amazing foods you can add to anything. I love it because it works. It adds to the weight loss boost, and its easy to add into recipes, juices, smoothies. It also contains everything you need for nutrient value and it's a great energy booster.

Loads of people throughout history have been on a quest to find the world's healthiest foods, and that is why we have "superfoods." There is one food that has stood out repeatedly, and this happens to be quinoa - for many great reasons.

Quinoa is not a grain of any type, and it is, in fact, **a seed**, so it contains no gluten. Such is the impact quinoa has had on the world, the United Nations has stated **it as a possible food to eradicate malnutrition and hunger**. One food can do this because it contains such a **broad spectrum of nutrients**, and for supply, it is **easy and cheap to cultivate.**

WHAT IS QUINOA?

Although the quinoa plant grows seeds rather than grains, they can be used in many of the same ways, and they are edible without much preparation. With the emergence of healthy lifestyles (the keto diet and paleo as prime examples), it was inevitable that quinoa would be included, and it is easy to see why. A seed that contains no gluten, yet is **power-packed with protein** and many other wonderful nutritional benefits. **What more could you ask for in a food?**

QUINOA NUTRITIONAL BENEFITS

Quinoa is what is called a **"complete protein source"** which is rare, no matter what foods you eat. To simplify this term, **quinoa contains all 20 amino acids** which **include the ten essential amino acids** (which the body is unable to produce on its own).

When you look at the benefits that quinoa brings, you can understand why it is the one food that should not be missed from your keto-styled/paleo-styled eating plan. It is remarkable for health and weight loss.

Promotion of Weight Loss – Because quinoa contains a high amount of insoluble fiber as well as protein, it gives that full feeling after a meal, especially when compared to refined grains. It also spreads energy for more extended periods, so you are less likely to peak and then crash, due to insulin levels fluctuating.

Quinoa also contains half of your daily recommended manganese levels. These stimulate hormones and digestive enzymes, as well. This makes it easier for the body to digest the other foods you eat. It really is an amazing food.

It's Gluten Free – Quinoa can be an excellent substitute in many recipes, and it is much healthier than other forms.

Other benefits see it helping in: the fight against cancers, aiding people with diabetes, and benefiting individuals who have cardiovascular illnesses. Another advantage of quinoa is its versatility, because you can add it to your juicing regime, green smoothies, in salads, or you can bake with it, and make healthy bars or cookies. So, slip in some quinoa to give you a much-needed protein and health boost. The weight loss potential is amazingly-awesome, too.

Scientific studies now confirm that quinoa is highly great for major benefits in overall health. The La Trobe University discovered that quinoa is great for reducing cardiovascular disease, and lowering cholesterol. The study also showed the metabolic syndrome was reduced which was a great finding, indeed. Metabolic syndrome is linked to type 2 diabetes, heart disease, stroke, and cardiovascular diseases. Weight loss was seen, and a 41% decrease was shown in both overweight and obese participants, when they added just 2.5 table-spoons on a daily basis.

SIX SUPER QUINOA RECIPES: BREAKFASTS:

RECIPE#1: PUMPKIN-QUINOA PANCAKES

This is full of flavor and so easy to do! I love this one. It's great for friends, too!

Ingredients

Dry Ingredients

- 3/4 of a cup of quinoa flour
- 1 teaspoon of pumpkin pie spice
- 1/2 of a teaspoon of cinnamon
- 1/2 of a teaspoon of baking soda
- 1/4 of a teaspoon of baking powder
- 1/4 of a teaspoon of real salt

Wet Ingredients

- 3/4 of a cup of pumpkin puree
- 1/2 a cup of Greek yogurt
- 1 tablespoon of molasses
- 1 tablespoon of maple syrup
- 3 tablespoons of almond milk
- 1 teaspoon of apple cider vinegar
- ½ a teaspoon of vanilla
- 2 eggs
- coconut oil (for cooking)
- your choice of honey and/or fruit, to taste

Instructions

- Combine dry ingredients in a medium bowl.
- Stir well and place aside.
- Combine wet ingredients (except the eggs) into a medium-sized bowl. Whisk well. In a separate bowl, whisk eggs, then stir them into the mixture.
- Place a skillet over medium heat. Add some coconut oil, no more than 1/2 a teaspoon. Let it melt, then add a ladle of the batter, about ½ a cup. Spread to make a pancake about 5" to 7" wide.
- Cook for approximately 3 minutes, or until bubbles start to appear. Flip and cook for another 3 minutes. Continue with the rest of the batter, adding more coconut oil, as required.
- Drizzle honey or fruit, to required taste.

RECIPE#2: YUMMY BANANA-QUINOA BITES

Bananas... need I say more? This is one of my favorite treats, because it tastes like homemade, and it is!

Ingredients

- 3/4 of a cup of whole wheat flour
- 2 teaspoons of baking powder
- a pinch of salt
- a pinch of baking soda
- 1 cup of cooked quinoa, cooled down
- 1 cup of mashed banana (2 to 3 medium bananas)
- 2 eggs
- 1/3 of a cup of almond milk
- 2 teaspoons of vanilla

Instructions

- Cook your quinoa.
- Preheat your oven to 180°C/355°F and grease a small cake tin.
- Combine your flour, baking powder, salt, baking soda, and the cooked quinoa.
- In a separate bowl, combine the banana, eggs, almond milk, and the vanilla.
- Mix your wet and dry ingredients by stirring well.
- Pour the mixture into your tin and place into the oven.
- Bake for 35-45 minutes, checking regularly.

Lunches:

RECIPE#3: AMAZING AVOCADO QUINOA

Full of nutrients with a scrumptious taste. I love how easy this one is. Even my nieces love these!

Ingredients

- 1 cup of arugula
- 1/2 a cup of cooked quinoa
- 1 cup of sautéed brussel sprouts
- 1/2 an avocado, sliced
- 1 teaspoon of olive oil (to cook brussels sprouts in)
- salt and pepper, to taste

Instructions

- Cook the quinoa.
- Sauté the brussel sprouts for approximately 15 minutes, or until lightly browned.
- In a large bowl, mix and toss together the arugula, the cooked quinoa, the sautéed brussels sprouts, and the avocado.
- Serve and enjoy.

RECIPE#4: BEAUTIFUL QUINOA CASSEROLE:

*This is homemade at its finest. You don't even feel like you are on
a diet... so, #winning!*

Ingredients

- 1 cup of quinoa
- 1 (10-ounce) can of mild, enchilada sauce
- 1 (4.5-ounce) can of chopped green chilis, drained
- 1/2 a cup of corn kernels, frozen, canned
- 1/2 a cup of canned black beans, drained and rinsed
- 2 tablespoons of chopped cilantro leaves
- 1/2 a teaspoon of cumin
- ½ a teaspoon of chili powder
- salt and ground black pepper, to taste
- 3/4 of a cup of shredded, low-fat cheese, divided
- 1 avocado, halved, seeded, peeled and diced
- 1 tomato, diced

Instructions

- In a large saucepan, use 2 cups of water to cook the quinoa.
- Preheat your oven to 380 degrees F.
- Oil a baking dish, or use nonstick spray to coat it.
- Now combine the quinoa, enchilada sauce, green chilis, corn, black beans, cilantro, cumin, and chili powder. Season with salt and pepper, to taste.
- Stir in the low-fat cheddar cheese.
- Spread quinoa mixture into the prepared baking dish. Top with a touch more cheese, as required.
- Place into oven and bake until cheese has melted, about 15 to 20 minutes.
- Garnish with the tomato and avocado.

Dinners:

RECIPE#5: SCRUMPTIOUS QUINOA MEATBALLS

*Italian inspired and yummy... this one is my ultimate favorite
because it tastes so good. Great for date night!*

Ingredients

- 1 lb. of ground turkey breast
- 3/4 of a cup of cooked quinoa
- 3 cloves of garlic, diced finely or minced
- 2 medium green onions, sliced thinly
- 1 egg
- 1 tablespoon of low-sodium soy sauce
- 2 teaspoons of sesame oil
- salt and black pepper, to taste
- 1/2 a teaspoon of sesame seeds

For the Sauce

- ¼ a cup of low-sodium soy sauce
- 2 tablespoons of rice wine vinegar
- 1 tablespoon of freshly grated ginger
- 1 tablespoon of honey
- 1 teaspoon of sesame oil
- 2 teaspoons of cornstarch

Instructions

- Preheat oven to 380 degrees F. Oil a large baking dish (you can
  coat with nonstick spray).

- In a large bowl, add ground turkey, cooked quinoa, minced garlic, onion, egg, low-sodium soy sauce, and the sesame oil.
- Add salt and pepper, to taste.
- Combine well with clean hands or a wooden mixing spoon.
- Form the mixture into 1 1/4 to 1 1/2-inch balls, it makes around 18-20 meatballs.
- Place meatballs onto your prepared baking dish then bake for 18-20 minutes, or until all the sides have browned and the meat is cooked all the way through.
- For the sauce: in a small saucepan, add together 1/2 a cup of water, low-sodium soy sauce, rice wine vinegar, minced ginger, honey, sesame oil, and stir until it's well mixed.
- In a small bowl, add cornstarch and 1 tablespoon of water. Add to the low-sodium soy sauce mixture and stir until thickened. This should take around 2 minutes.
- Garnish with the sesame seeds and green onion.

RECIPE#6: QUINOA AND BROCCOLI CASSEROLE

Again, it's just so yummy because it's homemade. Even kids love this one. A great way to hide the broccoli!

Ingredients

- 1 cup of uncooked quinoa
- 1 head of broccoli florets, finely chopped
- 2 tablespoons of virgin olive oil, divided into 2 parts
- 1/3 of a cup of breadcrumbs
- 3 chicken breasts, bones and skin removed, thinly-sliced
- salt and ground black pepper, to taste
- 2 tablespoons of butter, unsalted
- 2 tablespoons of all-purpose flour

- 2 cups of low-fat milk
- 1 and a 1/2 cups of low-fat cheddar cheese, grated and divided
- 1/3 of a cup of natural Greek yogurt

Instructions

- Preheat oven to 350 degrees F. Oil a large baking dish (you can coat with nonstick spray).
- In a large saucepan, add 2 cups of water and cook the quinoa as per the package instructions. In the last 5 minutes of cooking time, add chopped broccoli onto the top and steam until tender and cooked through.
- In a large pan, season your sliced chicken breasts with salt and pepper, adjust according to your taste.
- Place in skillet and cook, turn once, cook until cooked through, around 3-4 minutes each side. Cool before cutting into bite-sized pieces. Set aside.
- Melt butter in the skillet over a medium heat. Add flour and whisk until lightly browned, about 1 minute. Gradually add milk and whisk continually, then cook until slightly thickened, around 3-4 minutes.
- Add the quinoa, broccoli, chicken pieces, 1 cup of low-fat cheddar cheese, and the natural Greek yogurt. Season with salt and pepper, to your taste.
- Spread the broccoli mixture into the oiled baking dish and sprinkle on top (the remaining) 1/2 a cup of cheddar cheese.
- Place in the oven and bake until cheese melts, about 5 to 6 minutes.

For further information on losing weight with quinoa recipes check out my awesome book, "Top 50 Quinoa Recipes for Weight Loss and Optimum Health." Inside you'll discover the amazing benefits of quinoa, and why it's known as the most important food of our time. And, there's the top 50 quinoa recipes too; for breakfasts, lunches, and dinners! I'm sure you'll love this one! Click here! Another Free Ebook just for you!

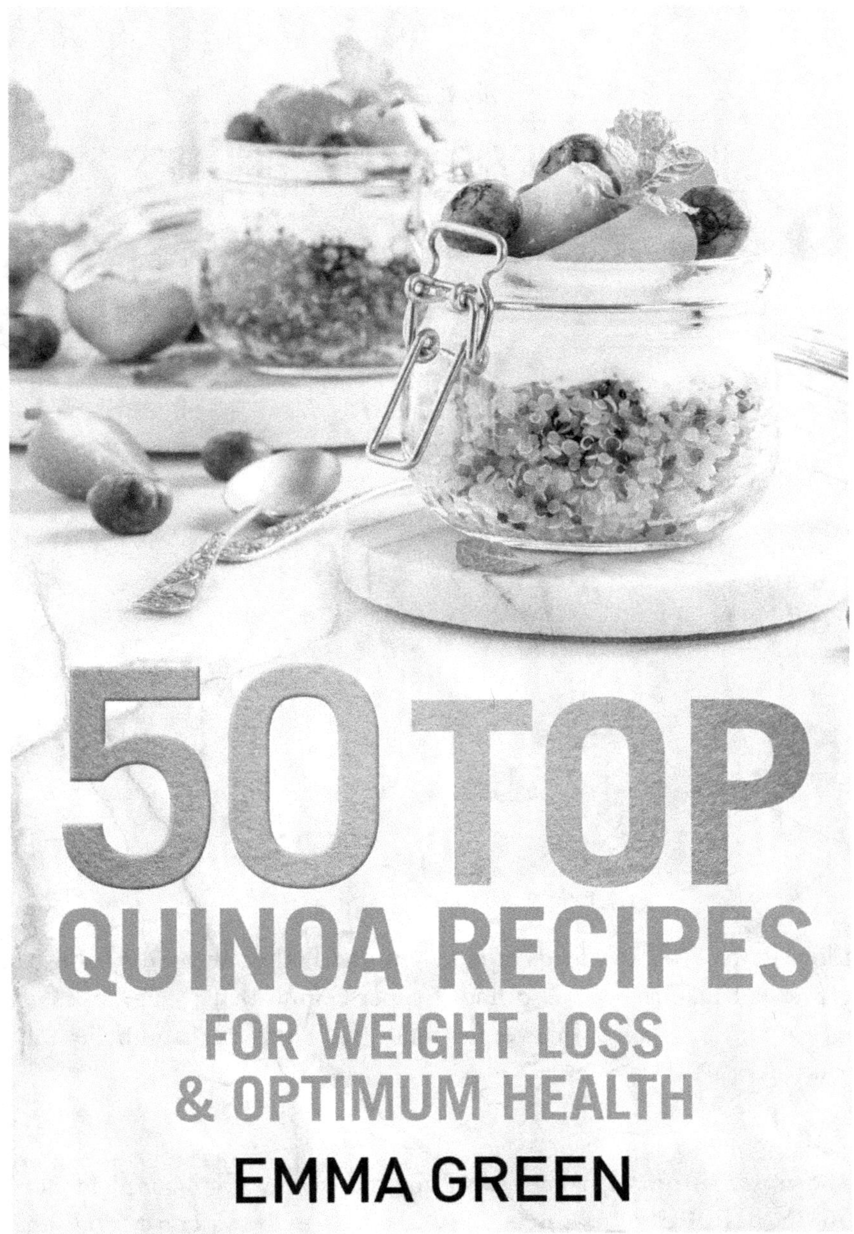

HERBS AND SUPERFOODS FOR WEIGHT LOSS

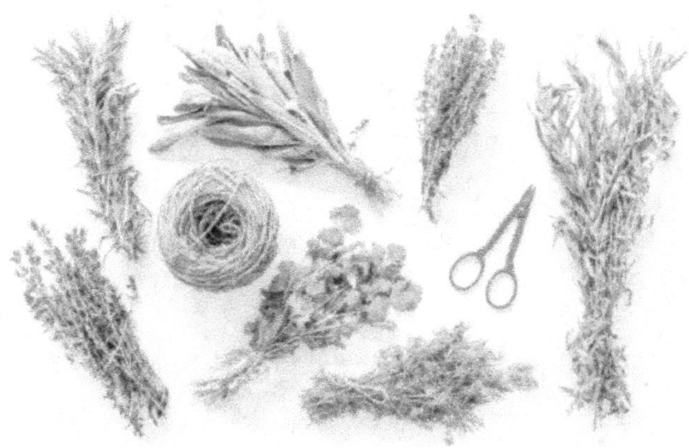

I love herbs, they give loads of nutrients and I adore the energy boost I get after I take them. I also find it super-helpful that I can add them into a tea, or a juice, or even a smoothie. They are so unbelievably versatile!

The **most important aspect** of any diet or nutrition supplementation **is definitely "balance."** As humans, we always crave food; not only because we get hungry, but because we have a need for it, to live. But if we give our body loads of one thing, and not another, it can become out of balance, and that's when the problems can arise. **Obesity, disease, feeling exhausted, not performing well, sleeping problems, and other imbalances become the forefront, without this balance.** Unfortunately, these small problems can skyrocket to massive ones, and then illness can eventually (and very unfortunately) lead to premature death.

The main factor is firstly, **the food we put into our body.** Because, in truth, this primarily needs to be metabolized by the body. And the body quite literally only has what you give to it. So, if you give it "junk," it will become "junk." It will perform and function **without real functionality, healing ability,** or **growth promotion** due to the lack of nutrients being provided. And this is when **we can get "sick" or "fat" or "out of balance."**

The second important factor is, **the absolute need for the body to ingest and absorb what it needs to use for its processes,** and **get rid of (and eliminate) what it doesn't require,** as waste products through sweating, urination, and via bowel movements.

THE THREE FACTORS NECESSARY FOR SUCCESSFUL WEIGHT LOSS AND BALANCE:

1. **It Really, Truly Does Matter What We Eat**
2. **We Need All Kinds of Foods for Balance**
3. **Diet Extremes Will Harm Your Health**

If health and weight loss are our overall goals, our focus must be on **maintaining a balance.** This is crucial. **When we create a nutritional balance, then weight loss can be achieved easily,** because the functions of the body can cope properly and maintain the actions that are necessary for the body to be at its best, peak performance level. **Optimum health promotes the weight loss we desire, over time.** This is a fundamental factor.

If we use a race car as a metaphor for our body, we can see a connection. Here the car's "food" is given as "fuel," and it is serviced regularly to keep peak performance. If you compare the body to a performance racing car, you can realize the need for good fuel as it pertains to overall performance. **The body craves great "fuel"** and when it is at its peak then it performs remarkably well. **This means that fat loss is achieved when the body is maintained well, and through the utilization of a balanced diet that contains a plethora of nutrients.**

A balanced diet is made up of **100 percent** in different foods. If we hold onto a regime to incorporate **20 percent salty foods, 20 percent sweet foods, 20 percent bitter foods, 20 percent spicy foods, and 20 percent sour foods,** then balance can be achieved. The basis of this balance is shown as highly relevant and viable in ancient Chinese nutritional practice, and it relates to the **Five Element Theory.** One that allowed Emperors to live for over a hundred years in China during the earliest dynasties. The principle allows the body to get lots of sources of nutrition that relate to different systems and organs within the entire body. Too much of one food will unbalance the process, and too little will do the same. Using the 100 percent rule for every meal, means that your body is taken care of in a harmonic balance. Do this for breakfast, lunch, and dinner, as a necessity. **Always have three meals a day at the same times.** Your body likes to know what's coming, and it will stay balanced more easily when you help it in this way.

**Your meals should always contain 20 percent from each group

mentioned, totaling 100 percent to create the perfect balance at each and every meal time. Remember, it's important, because each "group" pertains to a body system and function. Keeping balance allows the systems to keep theirs, too.

Great Salty Foods:

Butter, beef, beans, cheese, egg, fish, caviar, seaweed, soy sauce, tofu, ham, olives, processed foods, salt, and more.

Awesome Sweet Foods:

Almonds, bran, brazil nuts, cabbage, cakes, candy, canned fruits, carrots, corn, cream, eggplant, honey, ice cream, lettuce, milk, oatmeal, beans, cucumber, and more.

Fantastic Bitter Foods:

Asparagus, artichokes, bok choy, broccoli, celery, chocolate, cocoa, coffee, green vegetables, mushrooms, cabbage, tea, spirulina, cauliflower, and more.

Fantastic Spicy Foods:

Basil, cayenne pepper, chili, ginger, liquor, leek, garlic, dill, mustard, onions, oregano, parsley, pepper, thyme, wine, vanilla, and more.

Amazing Sour Foods:

Beef, bread, liver, raw fruit, sour cream, tomatoes, vinegar, yogurt, red meats, fresh water fish, mayonnaise, salad dressings, turkey, natural fruit juices, barbecue sauce, and more.

The importance of ingesting minerals, plants, and animals is detrimental to great health for nutritional purposes. **The aim is always to provide the prevention of illness and healing effects to the body,** so it can maintain a homeostasis (optimal cellular balance) and stay strong and healthy, for the long term. **When this happens, weight loss can be achieved** without any major stress on the body.

Over the course of history, our diets have had a primary focus that has seen food tasting great, looking great, and that it has functionality in terms of the way it ends up from the farm, to the store, and then finally on our dinner table. This is still important, **but many great superfoods and herbs have been negated over the centuries – and these are vital for weight loss and optimum health.**

Some of the pungent, more unusual herbs and superfoods were actually forgotten over time, and were actually even negated because of their unusual taste and smell, as well as the question pertaining to what they might be used for. But we can see how beneficial they can be. Let's have a look at some...

EXCELLENT SUPERFOODS AND HERBS TO ADD INTO YOUR DAILY REGIME

Please note: some herbs can have adverse side effects when taken alone or if too much is consumed at one time. But when taken in the right manner, they can do wonders, so always follow the guidelines with each herb you take.

"FANTASTIC!" GYNOSTEMMA: THE HISTORY:

The plant originates from China, Japan, Korea, and Vietnam. It was first discovered in the 1970s and was being used as an "immortality tea." It was (at this time) being tested as a sugar substitute, and it was then that all the health benefits it contained within it were found.

The plant consists of five leaves with serrated edges and belongs to the same family as the cucumber, yet it bears no fruit. Although relatively new, it has gained a lot of attention due to its benefits and antioxidant properties.

The Benefits and Scientific Evidence:

This plant has been shown to help bring the body back into balance in much the same way as ginseng. Tests show it contains four times the amount of saponins to that of ginseng and are called, "gypenosides." A number of these saponins convert to "ginsenosides" when consumed, so you have the benefits of both. When consumed, it helps the body's metabolic system to function well, and is also great for maintaining blood sugar levels because it can help to remove harmful blood fats.

The Negatives and Cautions:

Gynostemma, if used, should only be used for a continuous period of four months because it can have side effects such as nausea and increased bowel movements. It should also never be taken along with any medicines that are being used which affect blood clotting or suppression of the immune system. It should also be refrained from use if the individual is pregnant or breastfeeding.

How to Use:

The most common way for use is via a healthy tea. One spoonful of leaves to a cup of hot water and steep for fifteen minutes is enough to release all the beneficial compounds. It is also possible to find hot water extracts that have been converted to capsule form, for added convenience.

The Taste:

The tea has a slightly sweet taste which is much the same as green tea and nettle. Because it has strong, rejuvenating effects, it is commonly used as a replacement for coffee or caffeinated tea.

Source It:

Gynostemma comes under various names such as "Jiaogulan," "Miracle Tea," "Jiao Gu Lan," among others. When purchasing leaves for making tea, you should check they are organically grown because some have been found to contain traces of pesticides if non-organic. Also make sure no other additives are contained when purchasing.

"AMAZING!" CINNAMON: THE HISTORY:

Cinnamon has been used for thousands of years as a spice in cooking and also as a medicine. As time has gone on, the health benefits of cinnamon have been discovered, and now there is a lot of research that can support these medicinal claims.

The cinnamon we know is harvested by cutting stems on the "Cinnamomum" tree and removing the inner bark. These are the rolls/sticks we see before it gets processed and ground into the powder, and that we use on a daily basis.

The Benefits and Scientific Evidence:

Researchers have shown that from the most common herbs seen today, it is cinnamon that ranks number one as having the highest levels of protective antioxidants. Studies have shown that cinnamon helps the body's blood sugar levels to be maintained while also increasing insulin levels and increasing the metabolism of glucose.

Cinnamon is highly beneficial in weight loss because it has an influence on how sugar is metabolized in the body, and its transformation into fat. Another effect of cinnamon is it delays the passing of food from the stomach to the intestine, so you will feel fuller for longer, and for more extended periods of time.

The Negatives and Cautions:

If you use regular amounts in either capsule form or in drinks, it can be safe to be used while breastfeeding or while pregnant. More copious measures should not be taken because there is not enough scientific evidence on the effects of large quantities.

Cinnamon can also affect people with type 2 diabetes because it might lower their blood sugar level. This effect can also interfere with a person having surgery. If an individual was due to have an operation, they should refrain from taking any cinnamon two weeks before the surgery.

How to Use:

There are many ways to incorporate extra cinnamon into your diet. It can be added to herbal teas or sprinkled on cereals. It can also be added to your morning coffee and sprinkled onto smoothies. It is also possible to find it in capsule form for convenience. You can make your own healthy drink with one teaspoon of raw honey and one teaspoon of cinnamon in hot water.

The Taste:

Cinnamon has a spicy-sweet flavor and can be used as a way of reducing sugar levels when cooking. Compared to sugar (as a sweetener), cinnamon contains no calories per serving.

Source It:

There are two types of cinnamon available which contain all the health benefits, yet one brings more than the other. Ceylon cinnamon is referred to as "true cinnamon" and the other is known as cassia cinnamon, which is more than likely the one which you find in the supermarket. Organic Ceylon cinnamon can be found in health stores or ethnic markets.

"SUPERB!" GOJI BERRY: THE HISTORY:

The goji berry (aka lyceum fruit or wolfberry) is grown mainly in Tibet and northwestern China. The plant has vines which can grow to a length of fifteen feet which are full of the small red berries. The berry has been used throughout its history from the first-century Chinese writings, as a way to aid longevity.

The Benefits and Scientific Evidence:

For over five thousand years, the goji berry has been used to help boost the immune system, enhance the condition of the skin, and treat many other health concerns. A study in the Journal of Alternative and Complementary Medicine shows that the full benefits include: energy levels, mental awareness, overall healthier feelings, and less fatigue.

Widely considered a "superfood," they contain high levels of polysaccharides, vitamins, minerals, micronutrients, amino acids, and antioxidants (among others) - all without including high levels of fat or calories. It is the polysaccharides which are an excellent source of probiotic fiber that helps the body to digest food and make better use of the nutrients in other foods.

The Negatives and Cautions:

Consumption of goji berries can affect the following:

*Pregnancy and breastfeeding as they contain betaine which may lead to miscarriages.

*Allergic reactions if you are allergic to nuts, tomatoes, peaches, and/or tobacco.

*They can, in some cases, lower the blood pressure too much, so if you have low blood pressure or are taking medication for high blood pressure, they might be unsafe to consume. This is the same if you have diabetes, because your blood sugar levels might drop too low if you are on medication.

How to Use:

Goji berries can be eaten dried, made into a tea, or used in cooking. They can also be found in capsule form with the berries being in a dehydrated and powdered form.

The Taste:

The berries have a sweet and sour taste. If dried, they have a chewy texture much like raisins.

Source It:

Goji berries are easily found online or in health food stores, and in any of the forms mentioned above. They can also be bought in a juice form, yet for the full range of benefits, the berries should be made into fresh juice within forty-eight hours of purchase.

"WONDERFUL!" CHRYSANTHEMUM FLOWER: THE HISTORY:

The name "chrysanthemum" comes from the Greek words, "gold and flower." It was stated it was cultivated in China as early as 1500 B.C.

and was unknown to western cultures. Yet once it gained recognition and had been studied, it has since been used to help with weight loss, antiaging and increased blood flow. In Chinese medicine, it is still used to treat eye issues, inflammation, and poor circulation. Amazing cholesterol benefits have been shown with the use of chrysanthemum flowers. A recent study showed that even with high fat and cholesterol diets, there was a huge decrease in cholesterol levels shown in the participating groups. It's also well-known for its wonderful aid in digestion processes, its help in the absorption of food, its brain cell purifying abilities, and for its hormone adjustment capabilities. The chrysanthemum flower is truly beneficial in many ways.

The Benefits and Scientific Evidence:

Drinking chrysanthemum tea might bring many health benefits which can include heart health as a necessity, because it increases blood flow to the heart. It may also increase sensitivity toward insulin. Detoxification is improved as it targets heavy metals contained in the liver and helps them to be flushed from the body.

Chrysanthemum is naturally high in beta-carotene which is converted to vitamin A which can be helpful for eyesight. Other main areas affected are bone health and anemia. A significant boost to health is notable.

The Negatives and Cautions:

There is little evidence of the effects when drinking chrysanthemum tea while pregnant or breastfeeding, yet the main precautions come from anyone who has allergies toward plants of the same family. This includes daisies, marigolds, and ragweed, among others. Consuming chrysanthemum can cause the skin to show extra sensitivity to the sun.

How to Use:

Chrysanthemum is usually consumed as a refreshing herbal tea which can be drunk hot or cold. For weight loss, it is combined with other herbs to form fat burning formulas. It can be mixed with ginseng, lotus leaf, green tea, and Chinese honey locust, among others.

The Taste:

If consumed on its own, chrysanthemum has a mildly sweet taste, similar to honey. Yet if it's consumed as part of a fat burning tonic, it might have a mix of flavors of the green tea it can be mixed with, for example.

Source It:

Chrysanthemum can be quite easy to source and is available from many health food stores or Asian supermarkets. Organic varieties should be chosen to ensure no chemicals have been used in their growth. Prepackaged teas should also be avoided because they contain high sugar content.

"AWESOME!" ASTRAGALUS ROOT: THE HISTORY:

Astragalus is part of the same family as beans or legumes, and comes with a very long history of being used to boost the immune system and fight illness. Also known as milkvetch root and huang-qi, it can grow up to three feet in height and is native to north and east China.

Although there are over two thousand varieties of astragalus, only two are used for medicinal purposes, and these are astragalus membranaceus and astragalus mongholicus.

The Benefits and Scientific Evidence:

With scientific evidence backing it up, astragalus has been shown to have three components that help with health:

*Saponins: these lower cholesterol, boost the immune system, and help to prevent cancer.

*Polysaccharides: these contain anti-inflammatory benefits along with antiviral and antimicrobial properties.

*Flavonoids: these contain antioxidant properties and help fight free radicals, along with the ability for fighting heart disease, immunodeficiency viruses, and cancer.

The Negatives and Cautions:

Astragalus should not be used when pregnant or nursing, and anyone with an autoimmune illness should consult a professional before use. The following interactions can also occur with the following:

*Cyclophosphamide – this drug's effectiveness can be reduced.

*Immunosuppressant's – these drugs' effectiveness can be reduced. Many medications fall under this type. Always consult a professional.

*Lithium – unsafe levels of lithium in the body can occur if taken in conjunction with astragalus.

How to Use:

There are numerous ways you can take astragalus. It can be taken in capsule form, as a tincture, or (most commonly) dried and used to make a tea. The root can also be added to soups or stews. The powdered variety can also be mixed to produce a peanut butter alternative.

The Taste:

If used in soups or stews it adds a sweet, earthy flavor. This is the same as if it is made into a tea, and you can add a spoonful of honey to sweeten the taste a little. All you have to do is remove or strain the pieces as you would for tea leaves or a bay leaf, in cooking.

Source It:

It might be possible to find astragalus in Chinese supermarkets, yet it is widely available from many online companies in the root form or in capsule and root extract varieties. Make sure there are no nasty additives.

"EXCELLENT!" HE SHOU WU: THE HISTORY:

He shou wu is one of sixty superior tonic herbs out of ten thousand medicinal plants used in Chinese medicine, and where he shou wu (or fo-ti) is regarded as the best longevity tonic of them all. It has a long history in Chinese medicine in helping many of the body's vital organs. It has also been said it can raise vitality and sperm count, as well as maintaining a youthful look in a person's hair.

The Benefits and Scientific Evidence:

Studies that have been conducted show the cardiovascular system is improved by taking he shou wu, as well as helping to reduce hepatic fat in the liver. It can also be used to lift overall vitality and help with anti-aging as well as fortifying muscles, tendons, and the bones, too.

The Negatives and Cautions:

It is recommended not for use if an individual is pregnant or breast-feeding, or for the use of children under 5 years of age. Diabetics should also check first, as blood sugar levels might drop out of range.

Due to estrogen-like properties, anyone with hormone-sensitive conditions should refrain from taking it, in any dosage.

How to Use:

You can use he shou wu in the form of a tincture or as a fine powder that can easily be added and shaken in a juice or other drink. It is not ideal for tea because it is not soluble - so the full benefits will not be released. Another way is to use it is in capsule form.

The Taste:

The taste is an earthy and slightly salty taste, so it is better to mix it with something else, although a teaspoon of the powder can be taken with honey which can mask the flavor, if you are not keen.

Source It:

When purchasing, you should make sure that the roots are a minimum of four years old. You should also check that the roots have been cooked in the black bean method. If they have not been prepared via this technique, they will not contain the full range of benefits.

"PERFECT!" LICORICE: THE HISTORY:

Licorice is also known as "sweet root" for its use in making beverages and candies. It has also been used as a medicine for centuries. It is native to the Mediterranean and to Asia, and is classed as a weed.

The Benefits and Scientific Evidence:

Licorice root has benefits for gastrointestinal problems such as heartburn, stomach ulcers, and food poisoning. It also has immune boosting and anti-inflammatory properties thanks to the glycyrrhizic acid. Licorice can also help with respiratory problems, reducing stress levels, and protecting both the teeth and the skin. It also aids in cancer treatment. Licorice is also shown to help reduce sugar cravings. So, it's great for weight loss.

The Negatives and Cautions:

For licorice tea, you should not consume more than 8 ounces per day.

Other effects can be low levels of potassium which leads to hypokalemia. A study in 2012, showed anyone who ingested too much licorice in a period of two weeks experienced metabolism problems and fluid retention. Other negatives are high blood pressure and irregular heartbeat. Any form of licorice should be avoided by pregnant women or if they are breastfeeding.

How to Use:

Licorice can come in extract form and can be used as a sweetener in drinks, yet consumption should not exceed 30 mg per day for that use. Licorice can also be taken orally, as a capsule, and should not exceed 75 mg per day in that form.

If you use the leaves, these can be crushed and made into a tea. This has become popular, being sold and named, "Throat Coat Tea."

The Taste:

The taste can range in anything from sour or salty, to sweet and bitter, and it is quite pungent. It is one of the standard ingredients that is used in medicines to mask the real taste.

Source It:

Licorice can be found readily online via specialty retailers or in many health food stores. It is also possible to find the tea variety in larger supermarkets.

Some Other Super-Awesome Superfoods/Herbs Include:

- Ginseng Root
- Gotu Kola
- Acai Berries
- Jujube
- Cocoa
- Pine Pollen
- Colostrum
- Bone Broth
- Wheat Germ
- Organic Ghee
- Colloidal Gold
- Colloidal Silver
- Schizandra Extract
- Velvet Antler
- Reishi Mushroom

IN ADDITION TO HERBS AND SUPERFOODS

This list below, I would not consider superfoods, however, they are very healthy and should be considered in one's dietary plan for the nutritious and low-fat qualities that they share. They can be added into your diet to enhance your balance of foods in the **100 percent achievement rule**, where the **Five Element Theory** (discussed earlier) comes into play.

Remember, our diet needs balance, and **the more variety, the better**. As long as the benefits are healthy, tasty, nutritious, and great looking – you can't really go wrong. Each meal is made up of the sour, salty, bitter, sweet, and spicy elements in 20 percent equal parts. Thus, creating the **Five Element Theory** as a necessity, and for the whole body as a system that needs balance; every single day.

LET'S TAKE A LOOK THESE IMPORTANT INCORPORATIONS:

Fantastic Fish

Fish is full of protein and is a healthy, low-fat food that contains essential omega-3 fatty acids. Adding it to your diet can also help to lower blood cholesterol and definitively reduce the risk of cardiovascular disease. Baking is the healthiest way to cook fish without adding high amounts of other fats or oils to the meal.

Perfect Poultry

Poultry is one of the most beneficial proteins for good reason. It's lean, easily accessible, and has a very neutral flavor. Poultry is made up of many varieties of birds (domesticated ones). These types of poultry include: guineas, geese, chickens, pigeons, and turkeys.

A great tip is to cut the fat off before cooking. Always make sure you use a different cutting board for preparation than you do for the finished, cooked result. Many cases of food poisoning have occurred this way. It's also important to buy organic whenever possible. Never re-freeze poultry.

Awesome Organ Meats:

Organ meats are sometimes called "offal." The word offal comes from the term "off fall," which pertains to any part of an animal that falls away after butchery.

Liver, heart, kidneys, sweetbreads, brain, tongue, and tripe are all organ meats. Organ meats are sometimes called "superfoods" because they are fantastic sources of vitamins and nutrients, including: vitamin B, iron, phosphorus, magnesium, copper, vitamin A, vitamin D, vitamin K, and vitamin E and if cooked correctly you wouldn't even know you eating organs!

Wonderful, Healthy Vegetables:

It's important to include dark, leafy greens as well as tofu and ginger when you can. These healthy additions are full of antioxidants and contain imperative vitamins and minerals that are great boosts for health, and can aid in weight loss promotion, too.

Amazing Spinach – Great for its iron content, vitamin K, vitamin A, manganese, folate, magnesium, copper, vitamin B2, vitamin E, calcium, potassium, vitamin C, and vitamin B6.

Perfect Parsley – Well-known for its vitamin K, vitamin C, folate, iron, and vitamin A content. Contains flavonoids which are great for use as an anti-inflammatory. Parsley also helps to boost the immune system.

Terrific Kale – Helps with inflammation, detoxification, brain development in infants, vision health, supporting heart health, and helping to prevent cancer.

Beautiful Bok Choy – Aids bone health, heart health, and is an anti-inflammatory, and an immune booster. It's also great for skin health, and is also a fantastic blood pressure stabilizer.

Beneficial Collard Greens – A great source of vitamin B1, vitamin B6, iron, protein, copper, phosphorous, magnesium, vitamin B5, omega-3 fatty acids, folate, niacin, potassium, and vitamin B1.

Super Swiss Chard – Great for antioxidant boosting, blood sugar regulation, brain health, cancer prevention, blood health, and hair health.

Delicious Ginger – Fantastic for: nausea relief, digestive support, ulcer healing, immunity boosting, its anti-fungal qualities, pain reduction, cancer fighting, weight loss properties, anti-inflammatory properties, cholesterol lowering ability, and reducing arthritic pain.

Wonderful Tofu – Awesome for use as an alternative to red meat. A great source of protein. Also aids in weight loss promotion, and is great as a substitute for vegetarians who negate meat, nutritionally.

Superb Healthy Seeds:

Add seeds to meals, juices, or smoothies for more benefit. Include: **sesame seeds, chia seeds, flaxseeds, sunflower seeds, hemp hearts, pumpkin seeds, and wheat germ.**

Say "Yes" to Sesame Seeds – Copper, magnesium, and zinc.

Add Amazing Chia Seeds – Fiber, omega-3 fatty acids, protein, and antioxidants.

Up Your Intake with Flaxseeds – Omega-3, lignans, and fiber.

Add a Boost with Sunflower Seeds – Vitamin E, selenium, and magnesium.

Do Yourself a Favor with Hemp Hearts – Omega-3s and omega-6s.

Add in Pumpkin Seeds – Zinc, carbohydrates, anti-microbial properties, and antioxidants.

Don't Forget to Use Wheat Germ – Vitamin B1, vitamin B6, protein, and fiber.

For further information on losing weight with herbs and superfoods check out my awesome book, inside you'll discover the amazing benefits of some all-important herbs and superfoods, and the reasons why they're so important for health, detox, and weight loss. Click here!

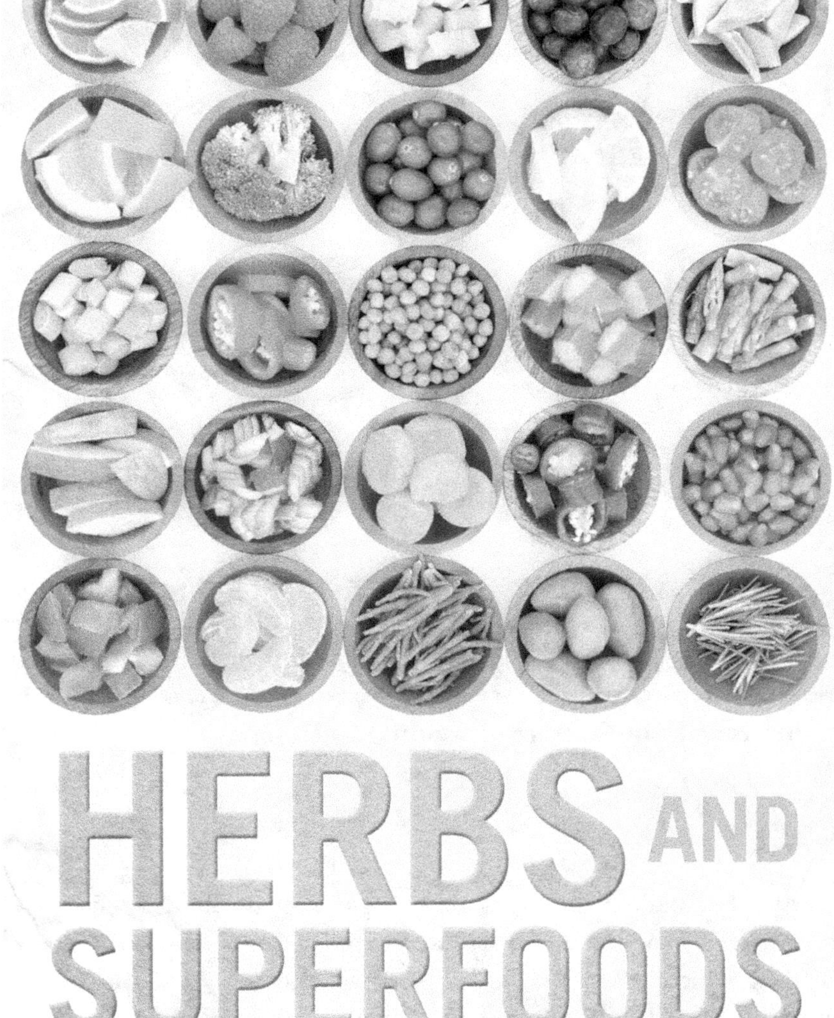

HERBS AND SUPERFOODS

FOR WEIGHT LOSS AND DETOX

EMMA GREEN

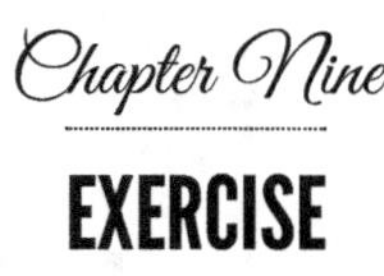

EXERCISE

Using exercise minimally is important for weight loss. But, we want to burn calories without putting excess strain onto the heart. **Yoga and meditation techniques are also wonderful for overall body maintenance and stress reduction.**

Sports

Sports are a fantastic way of losing weight because they never appear to be a regular workout. **Sports are fun** and bring out the competitive side which spurs you on that little bit more (with more calories burned). It might be the case that you are not that good at some sports, yet there are so many to choose from, and everyone has to start somewhere. **The secret is to make it enjoyable** - then burning those calories becomes a pleasure, not a chore.

Cardio Machines

Not everyone has the luxury of having a cardio machine at home, so the best way is to join a gym. These are great if the weather is bad, or you can fit in twenty minutes before work or after work.

Some of the More Common Machines:

Terrific Treadmills – These are not as good as free running, but they are enough to keep your heart rate up. Once you find a pace that is fast enough and pushes you to keep you sweating, you know you are on the right track!

Amazing Elliptical Trainer – These simulate the effects of skiing and give the whole body a workout. They are slightly behind a treadmill in the burning calorie stakes, but are great if you want a change - and something that is not as harsh on your feet or knees.

Awesome Stationary Bike – These are another great addition to cardio machines because you can push yourself and keep those calories tumbling. If your gym has an airbike, these are even better. The harder you push yourself, the harder the resistance. These can be a great way to end a workout, for even just five minutes.

Super-Fun Cross-Training

This is where several modes of exercise are used to develop a certain level of fitness. The types of training would vary between gyms, yet they have many benefits.

Enhanced Weight Loss Is One Benefit– Cross-training allows you to pick the exercises geared to weight loss and burning a specific number of calories. An excellent example is 30 minutes on an elliptical trainer and then stationary cycling for a further thirty minutes. Always stay within your own capacity for training.

Deliciously-Fun Dancing

There are many types of dancing classes you can join, yet the most famous is Zumba. So, if you want to raise that heart rate to the sounds of pumping Latin music, this can be just the thing to fit in some intense cardio and burn those calories.

Try and Double Up Over Time

It is essential to **pick exercises or sports you enjoy**, or use cross-training and Zumba to mix it up a little.

Here is an average of calories that can be burned for an individual, based on 160 lbs. in weight, as an example. **All of these exercises are based on one hour,** and you can mix and match and use them as part of your cross-training exercises for the week. **These activities are also based on moderate performance levels, rather than vigorous or light training schedules.**

Calories Burned Per Exercise Type:

- Outdoor Cycling – **600**
- Static Cycling Gym – **700**
- Stair Machine Gym – **1000**
- Rowing Machine Gym – **820**
- Elliptical Trainer Gym – **700**
- Aerobics – **500**

- Running – **800**
- Jogging - **700**
- Running up Stairs - **1200**
- Badminton – **320**
- Basketball – **450**
- Boxing Punch Bag – **450**
- Soccer – **680**
- Martial Arts – **800**
- Jump Rope – **800**
- Squash – **920**
- Beach Volleyball – **620**
- Kayaking – **380**
- Swimming, Freestyle – **550**
- Swimming, Butterfly – **850**
- Swimming, Leisurely – **450**
- General Housework – **250**
- Mowing the lawn – **450**
- Raking the Lawn – **330**
- Gardening – **300**
- Walking – **300**
- Zumba – **600**

Chapter Ten

THE BENEFITS OF JUICING FOR WEIGHT LOSS

The Importance of Cruciferous Vegetables

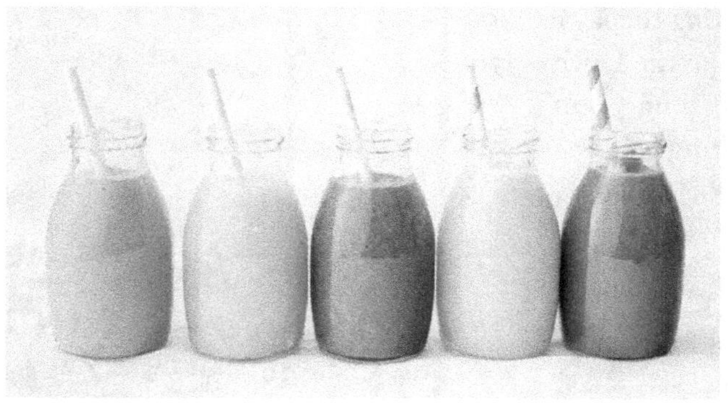

Cruciferous vegetables can be defined as: **vegetables in the Brassicaceae family**. Broccoli, cabbage, bok choy, and watercress are examples.

Thankfully, we are not helpless in our exposure to hormone-disrupting chemicals. The foods of the twenty-first century have been made up of many hormone-disrupting chemicals, unfortunately. And a good rule of thumb to remember is; if it comes in a packet and has additives of any kind, there's a good chance it's on the "no-go" list. So, blessedly, this is where the cruciferous vegetables list comes in. The big terms mentioned here are substances: **DIM (diindolylmethane) and I3C (indole-3-carbinol). All cruciferous vegetables are rich sources of these wonderful phytonutrients.** So, let's see what they do...

DIM (diindolylmethane) and I3C (indole-3-carbinol) can contribute to:

- Improving the Body's Metabolism
- Detoxification of the Entire Body
- Hormonal Balance Control in Men and Women
- Blood Sugar Level Control in Men and Women
- Reducing Inflammation in the Body, Overall
- Body Fat Reduction from Detoxification and Metabolism Improvement

Ultimately, these can mean **REAL** weight loss! Cruciferous vegetables also have their role in helping your body to **keep cancer away**. How amazing!

Cruciferous Vegetables List:

- Cauliflower (white or purple)
- Broccoli (green or purple)
- Brussel Sprouts
- Kale (green or purple)
- Bok Choy
- Cabbage (green, red or purple)
- Watercress
- Radish
- Broccoli sprouts
- Arugula (rocket)
- Kohlrabi (white or purple)
- Turnip
- Daikon

Juicing Recipes are Awesome for Weight Loss and a Healthy Digestive Tract

The whole cruciferous family are **spectacularly known for their soothing and healing effects on the digestive system.** A healthy digestive tract is of crucial importance when it comes to your absorption of vital nutrients. And so... just by using awesome juicing recipes that include cruciferous veggies, you will actually **improve the nutrient absorption capacity within your body,** and the ease (in terms of functionality) for your entire body as a whole.

Additionally, your juicer breaks down the added produce, so that your body can **assimilate the nutrients with functional ease.**

Tip: You can further increase the uptake of the nutrients by **adding a portioned amount of healthy fat when ingesting your juice.** This can be done in a number of ways. E.g. sprinkle some freshly ground flax or pumpkin seeds into the juice, as an example. Or, you could add some coconut, a slice of avocado, or an addition of peanut butter on a celery stalk.

SIX WONDERFUL JUICING RECIPES: RECIPE #1: RASPBERRY DELICIOUS

Fresh, tasty, and great in summer!

Ingredient List:

180g (1 whole) beetroot

40g (1/2 fruit) lemon

540g (3 medium) pears

120g (1 cup) raspberries

Directions:

Peel your lemon. You need to leave the skin on your pears. Chop up the lemon, beetroot and pears into cube-sized pieces. Just place the entire mix into your juicer. Blitz until silky, then shake and serve.

Helpful Tips: Add Liquid

Sometimes adding an inch or two of water is beneficial to aid in a smoother consistency, and for easier ingestion. Use rainwater or clean water. Not tap water, because it has loads of chemicals.

Amazing Facts: Water

Water makes up between 50-65% of the human body. This is dependent upon the size and leanness of an individual's tissue. Fatty tissue contains less water than lean tissue.

RECIPE #2: SMOOTH BLEND OF YUMMY: BEETROOT MAKES THIS ONE SO GOOD!

Ingredient List:

190g (1 medium) apple

180g (1 whole) beetroot

740g (12 medium) carrots

50g (1/2 fruit) lemon

270g (2 whole) oranges - peeled

Directions:

Peel orange, lemon, carrots, beetroot, and apple into larger-sized chunks. Place into your juicer, and let it blend until the mix is smooth. Serve icy cold with ice cubes if you want to.

Helpful Tips: A Powerful Juicer Is Paramount

Make sure you have a powerful juicer that's cleaned well and maintained properly. If not cleaned with hot water, bacteria can grow on its surface. It's important that health is always maintained where food is concerned.

Amazing Facts: Juicing Is Easy and Great for Health

Juicing can aid weight loss and health unbelievably when done properly. The ingredients used are paramount to the success. Fending off illness and longevity can also be achieved. Feeling amazing is the added bonus.

RECIPE #3: TOMMY TOMATO: TOMATOES ARE JUST SO FRESH AND GREAT TASTING!

Ingredient List:

1 tomato

1 cucumber

large handful cilantro

3 small zucchinis

2 celery sticks

Directions:

Chop vegetables. Add a cup of water if you have a blender because the fiber will be left in the mix. Blend until silky, and enjoy.

Helpful Tips: Nutrient Availability

Leave the skins on to provide even more nutrient availability. When you use the peel, you get more nutrient value. And you won't even know if it's well-blitzed.

Amazing Facts: Lovin' the Tomatoes

Tomatoes are beneficial for health because they aid in: prevention of cancer, skin maintenance, bone health, providing essential antioxidants, and are great for your heart. Wow!

RECIPE #4: LEMON-GINGER TINGLE: THIS ONE IS GREAT TO SHARE WITH A FRIEND!

Ingredient List:

1 bunch of cilantro

half head of bok choy

1 apple

squeeze of fresh lemon

1/4 teaspoon grated ginger

Directions:

Chop vegetables. Add a cup of water if you have a blender because the fiber will be left in the mix. Blend until silky, and enjoy.

Helpful Tips: Let the Kids Try

We all know how hard it is to keep our kids healthy, so let them help you and experiment with them in the kitchen. If we can get the next generation on board with healthy eating, we can help change the current trending statistics on a wider health scale.

Amazing Facts: Yummy Bok Choy

Bok choy is awesome for health. It aids in: bone health, heart health, inflammation, immunity, and skin health. Wow, loads of benefits there!

RECIPE #5: ITALIAN STALLION: PACKED FULL OF IRON, AND TASTES AWESOME!

Ingredient List:

1 bunch spinach

1 handful Italian parsley

1 cucumber

1 tomato

Directions:

Chop vegetables. Add a cup of water if you have a blender because the fiber will be left in the mix. Blend until silky, and enjoy.

Helpful Tips: Grow It

Growing parsley can be done easily. You don't need a big space or area and you can easily place it in a pot. Add it to everything. Parsley is a fundamental herb for human consumption.

Amazing Facts: Beneficial Parsley

Parsley has great benefits to health. This herb is amazing for strengthening immunity, and works on different aspects of the immune system. Parsley contains: vitamin C, vitamin A, vitamin K, folate, and niacin. A truly magnificent herb!

RECIPE #6: ORANGE AND RED TASTY: THE CARROTS AND BEETS TOGETHER, THEY ROCK!

Ingredient List:

180g (1 whole) beetroot

130g (2 medium) carrots

260g (2 whole) oranges

Directions:

Chop all ingredients and add them to your juice, together. Blend until smooth then serve cold. Add any garnish you like.

Helpful Tips: You Can Do Anything

The brain is very powerful. Did you know that you can do anything you want, especially when you believe it's possible? Yes, you definitely can. And I am here cheering you on, 100%, and all the way. Positivity helps a real-lot.

Amazing Facts: Marvelous Magnesium

Magnesium: known as the anti-stress mineral, it converts blood sugar to energy. Calcium: initiates DNA synthesis and helps bone health maintenance.

THE REAL BENEFITS OF GREEN SMOOTHIES FOR WEIGHT LOSS AND DETOX

The alkaline addition (through the use of smoothies) helps to not only get your body's **PH level back to where it should be**, but also works to maintain this for the long-term, as well.

Actually, **your PH level changes from hour to hour,** depending on the foods that you eat. **The meaning of PH is: Potential of Hydrogen**, and this is the measure of acidity or alkalinity within the body. You can use litmus paper to test it. You can buy it online and lick it to see your PH level. It changes throughout the day, and is dependent upon what you eat and drink.

It is important to understand, that when acidity in the body raises, the levels of minerals fall. So, you could see a level of between 5 and 7 when acidity takes over. **We want to aim for a PH of around 7.4 and upward**. But 7.4 is the magic number denoted by many studies and scientific findings related to health/healing and great internal balance.

Due to food being mass-industrialized over the last couple of hundred years, **food crops now contain less chloride, magnesium, and potassium, with increases in sodium,** unfortunately.

If you happen to be vegetarian or vegan, this methodology can easily work for you because the food contents are **nearly all vegetables and fruits. The recipes included here, have been adapted with weight loss and detoxification in mind.** Either way, you can add to them, because they are designed so that they are highly adaptable and useful for variation in tastes, so there is something there that will satisfy your appetite.

Add a nice snack to breakfasts, lunches, and dinners, and make sure your smoothie is the central appeal. I always tell people to make sure they add some meat, fish and protein (like chicken or pork). You want to achieve your goals safely, with health always in the forefront of your mind. Try and experiment with flavors and make balanced meals using the **Five Element Theory** as a rule of thumb. Smoothies can be a part of your day, for breakfast, lunch, and/or dinner.

The detox benefits of juicing include: the removal of toxins within the body, the prevention of digestion issues, it helps to combat weakness, bloating, mood swings, skin issues, and nausea. Other great reasons include: its liver cleansing ability, its energy boosting power, its reducing inflammation in the body ability, and the promotion of healthy, glowing skin.

For further information on losing weight with the help of juicing, check out my awesome book, "50 Juicing Recipes for Weight Loss and Healthy Living." Inside you'll discover the amazing benefits of some all-important juicing techniques, and the reasons why juicing raw food is so important for health and weight loss. You'll also get my most favorite juicing recipes that you can use on your all-important journey back to health. I'm sure you'll adore this one! Click here!

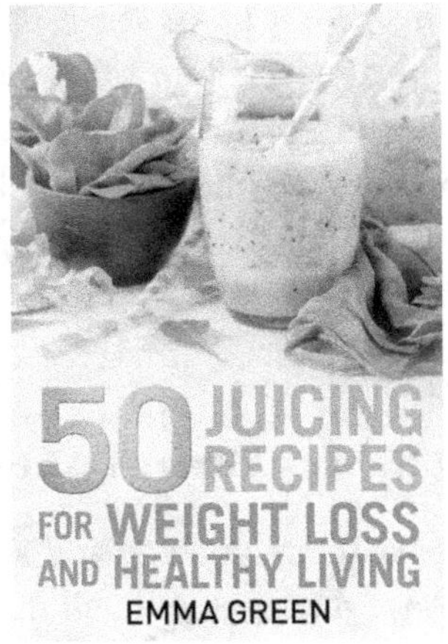

SIX AWESOME GREEN SMOOTHIE RECIPES: RECIPE #1: CHIA FREEDOM

Chia seeds are so good for me! I love the nutrition in this one!

Ingredient List:

2 oz. of collard greens

2 oranges - peeled

1 banana - peeled

1/4 of a cup of walnuts

1 tablespoon of chia seeds

1 cup of water

1 cup of ice

Directions:

When ready, simply process all the ingredients together in your favorite blender. You can shake it up or stir it up, then serve and enjoy. Cube or chop vegetables to make them blitz easier before blending. I like to add any leafy vegetables in last, and then add a touch more water if I want the consistency smoother or silkier. Great garnishes include: lemon, celery, chia seeds, or a slice of tomato. Add ice on a hot day to make the drink cooler.

Helpful Tips: Adding Rain or Filtered Water

To create a smoother consistency, you can add an inch or two of water. This will create a less dense mixture, and will make your juice easier to ingest.

Amazing Facts: Awesome Bananas and Oranges

Bananas and oranges are two of the most familiar smoothie elements, and this is for good reason. They blend beautifully into nearly any recipe, and provide a sweetness and creaminess that compliments the savory flavor of the greens. Bananas are full of potassium, and oranges add fiber and vitamin C.

RECIPE #2: WHEATGRASS WONDER: THE NUTS GIVE IT A BOOST, AND THE BANANA ADDS AMAZING FLAVOR!

Ingredient List:

1 1/2 oz. of Swiss chard

3 kiwis - peeled

1 banana - peeled

4 tablespoons of almonds

1 teaspoon of wheatgrass powder

1 cup of water

1 cup of ice

Directions:

When ready, simply process all the ingredients together in your favorite blender. You can shake it up or stir it up, then serve and enjoy. Cube or chop vegetables to make them blitz easier before blending. I like to add any leafy vegetables in last, and then add a touch more water if I want the consistency smoother or silkier. Great garnishes include: lemon, celery, chia seeds, or a slice of tomato. Add ice on a hot day to make the drink cooler.

Helpful Tips: Tips to Add in More

Smoothies are awesome because they allow you to add in protein powders and nuts or seeds as well. There is really no limit to what you can add. Go for it as long as it aids your health progression!

Amazing Facts: Wonderful Wheatgrass

One of the first superfoods to gain a lot of popularity was wheatgrass. The beauty of wheatgrass is that it contains chlorophyll, a green pigment in plants that has been shown to support the liver and is well-known to provide a boost of energy, over time.

RECIPE #3: COCONUT SPINACH WITH PEAR: COCONUT IS YUMMY FOR MY TUMMY!

Ingredient List:

1 1/2 oz. of baby spinach

2 pears - chopped

2 tablespoons of coconut flakes

1 tablespoon of hemp seeds

1 cup of water

1 cup of ice

Directions:

When ready, simply process all the ingredients together in your favorite blender. You can shake it up or stir it up, then serve and enjoy. Cube or chop vegetables to make them blitz easier before blending. I like to add any leafy vegetables in last, and then add a touch more water if I want the consistency smoother or silkier. Great garnishes include: lemon, celery, chia seeds, or a slice of tomato. Add ice on a hot day to make the drink cooler.

Helpful Tips: Blitz the Night Before

Smoothies are fantastic in terms of preparation and ease. You can prepare them in the evening and refrigerate the jug, drinking the blitzed recipe in the morning, and therefore, letting the flavors permeate overnight. If you do this, you won't need to add ice to your recipe, though. Yummy!

Amazing Facts: Coconut Flakes and Hemp Seeds Rock

Coconut flakes and hemp seeds add inflammation-lowering omega-3 fatty acids. Omega-3 is used to help the body lower the risk of heart disease, depression, arthritis, and dementia. Your body can't make omega-3, it needs to be added to the diet.

RECIPE #4: SUNFLOWER SPINACH

Sunflowers have loads of benefits, and the iron from the spinach is here too! what types of benefits?

Ingredient List:

1 1/2 oz. of baby spinach

1 banana - peeled

1 tablespoon of sunflower seeds

1 teaspoon of cinnamon

1 cup of water

1 cup of ice

Directions:

When ready, simply process all the ingredients together in your favorite blender. You can shake it up or stir it up, then serve and enjoy. Cube or chop vegetables to make them blitz easier before blending. I like to add any leafy vegetables in last, and then add a touch more water if I want the consistency smoother or silkier. Great garnishes include: lemon, celery, chia seeds, or a slice of tomato. Add ice on a hot day to make the drink cooler.

Helpful Tips: Add a Snack Too

For breakfast and lunch, you can make your favorite smoothie and just add a snack to make it a combo to aid in weight loss. Try grilling fish, or eating a lean pork, chicken or another healthy addition.

Amazing Facts: A Combined Goodness Here

Cinnamon is great as an anti-inflammatory. Spinach is full of vitamins, and the apples add both antioxidants and fiber to the recipe. The banana is great to get potassium and magnesium from, and the sunflower seeds have omega-3s. Wow!

RECIPE #5: PINEAPPLE-SPINACH FANTASY: PINEAPPLE... #WINNING! CHANGE

Ingredient List:

1 1/2 oz. baby spinach

4 oz. pineapple - chopped

1 persimmon - chopped

3 tablespoon of coconut flakes

2 tablespoons of dried mulberries

1 cup of water

1 cup of ice

Directions:

When ready, simply process all the ingredients together in your favorite blender. You can shake it up or stir it up, then serve and enjoy. Cube or chop vegetables to make them blitz easier before blending. I like to add any leafy vegetables in last, and then add a touch more water if I want the consistency smoother or silkier. Great garnishes include: lemon, celery, chia seeds, or a slice of tomato. Add ice on a hot day to make the drink cooler.

Helpful Tips: Top the Persimmons

Take the tops off of the persimmon and the pineapple first, to aid in ease when chopping.

Amazing Facts: Mulberries are Super-Cool

Native to China, mulberries are mildly sweet and contain a very high amount of vitamin C, fiber, and much-needed potassium as well. Additionally, they contain iron, which is needed by the hemoglobin in red blood cells because of its ability to bind with oxygen, and consequently transport it throughout the body.

RECIPE #6: YUMMY CHAI: THIS IS MY ALL-TIME FAVORITE BECAUSE IT HAS EVERYTHING I LOVE!

Ingredient List:

1 1/2 oz. of baby spinach

5 oz. of butternut squash

1 banana - peeled

1/2 teaspoon of chai spice

4 tablespoons of almonds

1 cup of water

1 cup of ice

Directions:

When ready, simply process all the ingredients together in your favorite blender. You can shake it up or stir it up, then serve and enjoy. Cube or chop vegetables to make them blitz easier before blending. I like to add any leafy vegetables in last, and then add a touch more water if I want the consistency smoother or silkier. Great garnishes include: lemon, celery, chia seeds, or a slice of tomato. Add ice on a hot day to make the drink cooler.

Helpful Tips: Keep it Cool or Not

Every smoothie recipe can be iced or left at room temperature if the weather isn't warm enough to drink it cool. The best thing about smoothies is you have so many choices. With flavors, combinations and add-ons! It's only limited by your imagination...

Amazing Facts: Almond Milk and Chai Spices Are Perfect

Almond milk and chai spices create the perfect chai-latte effect. In essence, you have all the flavor of a delicious milkshake with a super-duper nutritional punch.

For further information on losing weight with green smoothies, check out my amazing book, "50 Green Smoothie Recipes for Weight Loss and Detox." Inside you'll discover the amazing benefits of raw foods, and the reasons why they're so important for health, detox, and weight loss as the main focus points. Includes 50 awesome recipes you can use each day! I'm super-sure you'll get loads of information and usage from this one! Click here!

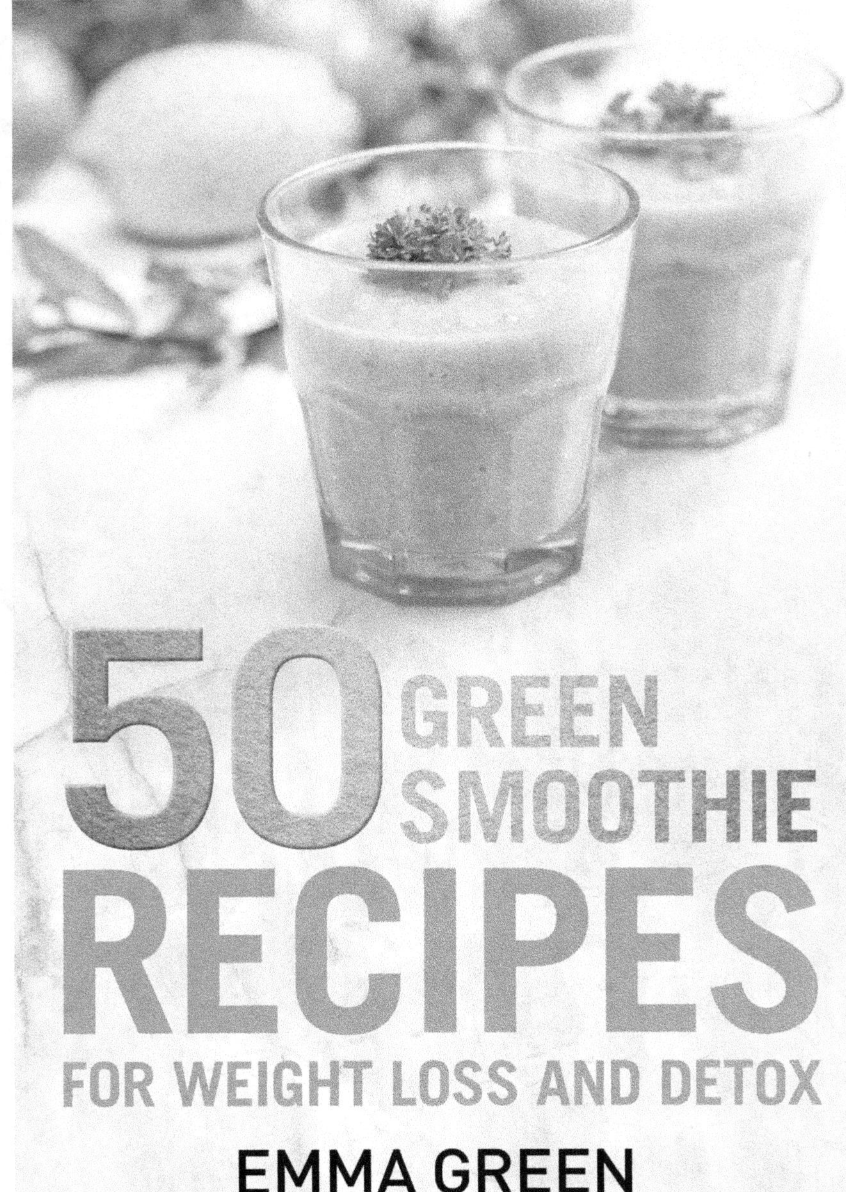
50 GREEN SMOOTHIE RECIPES
FOR WEIGHT LOSS AND DETOX
EMMA GREEN

IN CONCLUSION

Some of the big issues caused by being overweight or obese include: diabetes, cardiovascular disease, arthritis, stroke, and depression, and many more. Usually complications arising from those things. In addition to losing weight for health, you will increase your energy levels, build your self-esteem, and your social capacity should grow because you'll feel so much better from doing it.

My life has been lifted skyward since I lost weight. I feel better, look better, have loads more energy, and can truly say that I love life again. And, I can tell you, I never thought I'd ever say that. And you can too! It can take time, but it's definitely worth it, and you will increase your overall health, too! And that's a major, super-important plus.

Thank you for joining me here! I know you can do this... because I did. When you have read through all the chapters, you will see that each area is separate, and once you have read it all, you then have to piece together your own, individual plan. This task of losing weight is not easy, yet nothing worth doing, ever is.

By pulling together the very best ways of **cutting out the junk**, and helping your body to perform at its best, you can lose weight.

With the inclusion of following the **keto and paleo diet eating styles**, your body will fall into a state of ketosis - and you will be burning fat while resting. Losing lots of weight would not be possible if it was not for this state that the body falls into. **The 6 cups per day rule is also a much-needed practice. Add in juicing and green smoothies, the paleo and keto recipes, superfoods/herbs, then the exercise needed to burn the stated calories,** and if you want to shed the weight a little more quickly.

Hard work always pays off if you do things correctly. **Plan your week** and stick to what you have planned, and you **WILL** get results. Each area works together with the other, and they are all geared to you losing weight and leading a much healthier lifestyle on the whole. And this promotes health now, and in the future.

As usual, I am sending you all the luck in the whole, wide world, and I'm always here, cheering you on! I know you've got this! You are so worth it.

I am sending you loads of love, and my wishes for the best of luck in your weight loss journey. Lots of love, always, *Emma* xx

P.S. You've totally got this!!!